W9-BZX-089

BASIC CONCEPTS IN
MEDICAL
GENETICS

. . . .

Notice

Medicine is an ever-changing science. As new research and clinical experience broaden our knowledge, changes in treatment and drug therapy are required. The author and the publisher of this work have checked with sources believed to be reliable in their efforts to provide information that is complete and generally in accord with the standards accepted at the time of publication. However, in view of the possibility of human error or changes in medical sciences, neither the authors nor the publisher nor any other party who has been involved in the preparation or publication of this work warrants that the information contained herein is in every respect accurate or complete, and they are not responsible for any errors or omissions or for the results obtained from use of such information. Readers are encouraged to confirm the information contained herein with other sources. For example and in particular, readers are advised to check the product information sheet included in the package of each drug they plan to administer to be certain that the information contained in this book is accurate and that changes have not been made in the recommended dose or in the contraindications for administration. This recommendation is of particular importance in connection with new or infrequently used drugs.

BASIC CONCEPTS IN
MEDICAL GENETICS

A STUDENT'S SURVIVAL GUIDE

Marshall Horwitz, M.D., Ph.D.
Division of Medical Genetics
Department of Medicine
University of Washington School of Medicine
Seattle, Washington

With contributions from (Chap. 7, Cytogenetics):
Mary Beth Dinulos, M.D.
Division of Medical Genetics
Department of Pediatrics
Children's Hospital Medical Center
University of Washington School of Medicine
Seattle, Washington

Illustrations
Kris Carroll
Bainbridge Island, Washington

Series Editor
Hiram F. Gilbert, Ph.D.

DES PLAINES PUBLIC LIBRARY
1501 ELLINWOOD STREET
DES PLAINES, IL 60016

McGraw-Hill
Health Professions Division
New York   St. Louis   San Francisco
Auckland   Bogotá   Caracas   Lisbon   London   Madrid
Mexico City   Milan   Montreal   New Delhi   San Juan
Singapore   Sydney   Tokyo   Toronto

McGraw-Hill

A Division of The McGraw·Hill Companies

BASIC CONCEPTS IN MEDICAL GENETICS:
A STUDENT'S SURVIVAL GUIDE

Copyright © 2000 by The McGraw-Hill Companies, Inc. All rights reserved. Printed in the United States of America. Except as permitted under the United States Copyright Act of 1976, no part of this publication may be reproduced or distributed in any form or by any means, or stored in a database or retrieval system, without the prior written permission of the publisher.

1234567890 DOCDOC 09876543210

ISBN 0-07-134500-0

This book was set in Times Roman by Better Graphics, Inc. The editors were Stephen Zollo, Janet Foltin, Susan R. Noujaim, and Peter J. Boyle; the series editor is Hiram F. Gilbert, Ph.D.; the production supervisor was Catherine Saggese; the cover designer was Mary McDonnell; the index was prepared by Barbara Littlewood. R. R. Donnelley and Sons Company was printer and binder.

This book is printed on acid-free paper.

Library of Congress Cataloging-in-Publication Data

Basic concepts in genetics: a student's survival guide / editor, Marshall Horwitz.
    p. cm.
   ISBN 0-07-134500-0.
   1. Genetics.   2. Medical genetics. I. Horwitz, Marshall.
   [DNLM: 1. Genetics, Medical. QZ 50 B3107 2000]
QH430 .B38   2000
616'.042--dc21   99-053279
                                     CIP

· C O N T E N T S ·

BASIC CONCEPTS IN
MEDICAL
GENETICS

· · · · · · · · · · ·

· C H A P T E R · 1 ·

INTRODUCTION

·

Sometime early in the twenty-first century—probably before you finish medical school—the human genome will be sequenced in its entirety. The three billion basepairs of the haploid human genome represent about the same amount of data as encoded in just a single CD-ROM. It is indeed mind boggling to consider the fact that so little software can encode the designs for such a complicated machine, chiefly, a human being.

But rather than reducing humanity to such a statistic, we prefer to turn the fact on its head and note that humans accomplish at least one feat that no computer will for quite some time: we can take a CD-ROM worth of information and squeeze it into the confines of a tiny cell with volume that is less than what a CD takes to store just a single bit of information. Given that there are about a trillion cells in a human being, each containing a complete copy of the human genome in itself, our bodies enshrine and manage unfathomable volumes of data. Yet a change in as little as just a single bit (one basepair), if one is unlucky, can give rise to cancer or a new mutation responsible for an inherited disease. The fact that this process works so well, for most of us, most of the time, is testimony to just how remarkably elegant the human machine is.

But, of course, things do go wrong sometimes. The DNA mutates, the information is lost or scrambled, and the result is a genetic disease, whose legacy may be continued inheritance in a family's lineage for untold future generations, or, of even more immediate concern to that person, a life-ending malignancy. Understanding human heredity and how it relates to disease is the goal of this text.

Current statistics offer a compelling argument for the role of a course in genetics in contemporary medical education. Genetics issues are present at every stage of life.

About 50% of all first trimester spontaneous abortions result from a chromosomal abnormality. About 3% of all newborns have a major genetic disease. About a third of all pediatric hospital admissions are the result of

1

genetic disease. About half of all pediatric deaths are ultimately attributable to genetic disease. About 2% of all adults will suffer from a single gene genetic disease. The vast majority of common diseases like diabetes mellitus, atherosclerotic vascular disease, and mental illness are the result of the additive effects of genes conferring variable degrees of risk interacting with the environment.

Times are changing fast enough that a working knowledge of the basics of human genetics are most likely to factor even more prominently in any physician's career from our present time onward.

We might like to entitle this book *Human Genetics for Dummies*. We cannot because the publisher of that popular line of books would not allow it. But, we also should not. That is because this material is sufficiently complicated and fast-changing enough that it is a difficult topic for anyone to comprehend. Indeed, one recent study found that physicians in practice incorrectly ordered a genetic test predicting colon cancer about one-half of the time and misinterpreted the results of that test about a third of the time. For a test designed to give a discrete answer, this sort of incompetence renders such a powerful test virtually meaningless or, even worse, downright dangerously misleading. Imagine the consequences of falsely reassuring someone that they are not likely to inherit cancer, or, of mistakenly leading an individual to believe that they will inherit cancer. Such false counsel can have profound influences on the decisions one will make in life: if one will marry and have children, whether one will continue to seek employment, or even if one will choose to end his or her life. As genetic tests become more ubiquitous and more complicated, the potential for misinterpretation of tests becomes even greater. There is also the problem of misapplication of correctly interpreted tests; as a society, we have yet to come to grips with the consequences of such testing. It is, therefore, an imperative that the modern physician become fully versed in this stuff.

This book is intended to be a reasonably complete synthesis of fundamental genetic principles illustrated with clinical examples, and one that can be read in a single, long sitting. It is an outgrowth of the syllabus used to teach medical genetics to second year medical students at the University of Washington, in a 22-hour course comprised of lecture and small group problem-based learning.

This text benefits from the contributions that numerous faculty members and fellows have made to the course over the years. We gratefully acknowledge these individuals, many of whom were our own teachers: Arno Motulsky, George Stamatoyannopoulos, Roberta Pagon, Wylie Burke, Peter Byers, Ron Scott, James Evans, Thomas Bird, Virginia Sybert, Louanne Hudgins, Edith Cheng, Kathy Leppig, Robin Bennett, Michael Raff, Hanlee Ji, Mark Hannibal, Melissa

Parisi, Mark Nuñez, Albert La Spada, Mark Kay, David Schowalter, David Russell, and Karen Swisshelm. We owe special thanks to Gail Jarvik, whose lectures on complex traits served as the basis for the organization and examples in Chapter 8. Many more fellows and faculty have further contributed to the implementation of the course and the evolution of the approach to medical genetics in Seattle, and we regret that the list is too long to print here.

We also wish to thank the editorial staff at McGraw-Hill, including Jim Morgan, Peter Boyle, Janet Foltin, and Susan Noujaim. Hiram Gilbert of the Baylor College of Medicine, and author of the biochemistry text in the series, further provided valuable advice.

GENES, CHROMOSOMES, AND MEIOSIS

•

• • • • • • • • • • • •

DEFINITION OF A GENE

Gene: The basic hereditary unit, initially defined by phenotype. By molecular definition, a DNA sequence required for production of a functional product, usually a protein, but rarely, an untranslated RNA.

Genotype: An individual's genetic constitution, either collectively at all loci or more typically, at a single locus.

Phenotype: Observable expression of genotype as a trait or disease.

Allele: One of the alternate versions of a gene present in a population.

Locus: Literally, a "place" on a chromosome or DNA molecule. Used fairly interchangeably with "gene" and sometimes used to refer to a collection of closely spaced genes.

Genes were originally defined by Mendel, a nineteenth century Austrian monk who formulated the basic rules of inheritance based on observations and experimentation in pea plants. Mendel defined genes as the theoretical unit responsible for an observable property of an organism. We call this property a "phenotype." In animal genetics, and particularly medical genetics, phenotype has a rather pejorative connotation and is usually used with reference to some defect or disease. Mendel began his studies by observing how flower color, seed shape, and other simple properties of pea plants were inherited. He correctly deduced that each parent contributes one copy of a gene for a particular trait, but that there were different versions of a gene, or "alleles," within a population. Some of these alleles function "dominantly," in that they are sufficient to cause the particular phenotype regardless of the allele contributed by the other parent. Other alleles act "recessively" and require that the opposite parent contribute a similar allele for the phenotype to be manifest. We will come back to a discussion of mendelian segregation patterns later and see how these simple concepts, first elaborated in plants, are equally applicable to human genetic disease, even in this era of profound knowledge of the molecular properties of a gene.

A gene corresponds to a physical location, or "locus," along a chromosome that relates to a particular sequence in a DNA molecule.

THE CENTRAL DOGMA

What is termed the "central dogma" of molecular biology and genetics is the fact that a gene is chemically encoded in DNA, that the DNA is "transcribed" into a working RNA copy, and that the RNA is "translated" into a protein, which, in turn, is molecularly responsible for effecting the phenotype.

DNA

Mendel and other early geneticists developed a sophisticated genetic model without knowledge of the physical basis of the gene. It is, therefore, not the intention of this book to comprehensively review biochemical aspects of genetics. Nevertheless, a simple review of some molecular genetics principles makes both of our jobs easier. The physical basis of the gene is DNA. The three components of a DNA molecule are the phosphodiester backbone, the chemical base, and the carbohydrate unit, deoxyribose, which attaches the two together. There are four different DNA bases. Adenine (A) and guanine (G) are purines, distinguished by two rings, whereas thymine (T) and cytosine (C) are single ringed pyrimidines. DNA usually is comprised of two strands intertwined in a double helix that are held together by complementary basepairs. A purine basepairs with a pyrimidine. Thus, A pairs with T, while C pairs with G. Each chromosome is one long DNA molecule. Since each strand of the DNA molecule is held to the other DNA molecule by non-covalent bonds, a DNA molecule may be separated into its two component strands.

RNA

The DNA encoding a gene is transcribed into temporary messenger RNA (mRNA) copies whose function is limited to translation into protein. RNA is similar to DNA, with a few exceptions. First, it is generally single stranded. A single molecule can, and usually does, fold back onto itself to form complicated secondary and tertiary structures, however. Second, in the place of thymine, RNA uses the base uracil (U). Third, the carbohydrate base of RNA, ribose, contains an extra hydroxyl group at the 2' position. Like DNA polymerase, RNA polymerase synthesizes DNA in a 5' to 3' direction. The primary transcript is made in the nucleus; it is edited to remove "introns," sequences that do not code for proteins and that are vestiges of a gene's evolutionary history, then transported to the cytoplasm for translation into polypeptides.

All DNA and RNA polymerases synthesize nucleic acids in a 5' to 3' direction.

PROTEINS

Proteins are polypeptides composed of amino acid building blocks. Twenty different amino acids are used in protein synthesis. During translation on the ribosome in the cytoplasm, the RNA sequence is read in three base "codons." There are 64 possible triplet codons. Since there are just 20 amino acids, each amino acid is represented by one or more of the possible triplet codons, and the code is redundant in this regard. Proteins are then synthesized amino terminal to carboxyl terminal until one of three "stop codons" is encountered. At that point, polypeptide chain synthesis terminates, and the protein is released from the ribosome. The protein may then be post-translationally modified with glycosylation or other processes and then sorted to the appropriate intracellular compartment or secreted into the extracellular environment.

Proteins are synthesized from amino terminus (N) to carboxyl terminus (C).

THE BASIC STRUCTURE OF A GENE

All genes have the same basic components (Fig. 2-1). The 5' region contains "promoter" and "enhancer" elements, which are responsible for punctuating the start of a gene and recruiting the binding of RNA polymerase and other transcription factors. Next, comes the ribosome binding site. This part is transcribed and serves to allow recognition of the mRNA by the ribosome for ultimate translation into a protein. Shortly behind the ribosome binding site is the ATG initiation codon (actually AUG in the mRNA), encoding a methionine residue. Most human genes are interrupted by introns, sequences that do not contribute information to the gene and that must be excised before the transcript matures and is exported to the cytoplasm for translation. At the end of the coding sequence is one of three termination codons (TAA, TAG, TGA—UAA, UAG, and UGA, respectively, in the mRNA). The 3' region contains a "polyadenylation" signal that is recognized by enzymes that attach a polyA tail to the mature mRNA.

Eukaryotic mRNA, such as in humans, differs from prokaryotic mRNA by the presence of a 5' chemical modification known as the "CAP" site, introns in the immature nuclear transcript, and a 3' polyA tail. Eukaryotic genes encoding proteins are transcribed by RNA polymerase II.

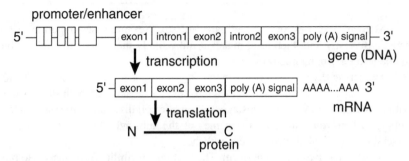

Figure 2-1   Molecular aspects of the central dogma.

DEFINITION OF A CHROMOSOME

CHROMOSOME VERSUS CHROMATID

Chromosome: A single DNA molecule condensed on a protein scaffold in the nucleus of a cell. Each chromosome contains thousands of genes (Fig. 2-2). Humans have 22 pairs of "autosomes" and one pair of sex chromosomes (X and Y), for a total of 46.

Chromatid: One of two identical parallel DNA strands in a mitotic cell following DNA replication.

Why do we need chromosomes? DNA is a long, thin flexible molecule. The extended length of the human genome would reach several meters unless there were a means for compactly folding and organizing the DNA to fit within the confines of a cell.

MEIOSIS

Meiosis: Addresses the problem of preventing genome size from doubling at each generation in a sexual organism. It is the cell division process in which "haploid" gametes are formed from "diploid" germ cells. Mistakes in meiosis are responsible for major chromosomal abnormalities. It is also the time when "recombination" between each parental chromosome homolog takes place.

Meiosis (Fig. 2-3) is part and parcel of sex. Sex increases opportunity for genetic diversity and, therefore, makes it more likely that a species will be able to adapt to environmental pressures.

Meiosis is divided into two general stages, meiosis I and meiosis II. Meiosis I and meiosis II are then subdivided into several substages, which share names with each other and with the substages of somatic cell division (mitosis). It is less important that you remember the names of the substages than gain an overall understanding of what meiosis accomplishes.

Meiosis has two jobs to perform. The first responsibility of meiosis is to prevent a doubling in the quantity of chromosomes from one generation to the next. Just imagine what would happen if the "germ cells" (sperm and egg) had the same chromosomal content as "somatic cells" (every other type of cells except

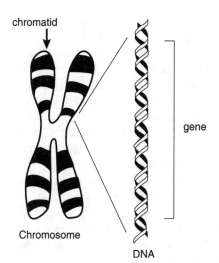

chromatid

gene

Chromosome

DNA

Figure 2-2   Chromosome, chromatid, gene, and DNA.

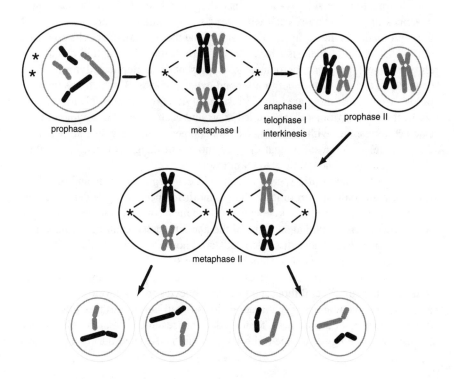

prophase I

metaphase I

anaphase I
telophase I
interkinesis

prophase II

metaphase II

Figure 2-3   Male meiosis.

for the germ cells). The number of chromosomes would double at fertilization, and children would have a genome twice as big as their parents.

In every pair of chromosomes in every individual, one chromosome came from the mother and the other from the father. Normally, the chromosomes are not microscopically visible in a cell. Only during mitosis and meiosis do the chromosomes condense and become microscopically visible in order to facilitate their mitotic or meiotic segregation. During the formation of an egg or a sperm, one parental chromosome from each pair is randomly picked for inclusion in the gamete. The way that this is accomplished is that the 23 pairs of chromosomes actually form a physical pair (called a synapse) and then line up along the midline of the cell. Each pair lines up in a random orientation, so that in one pair the chromosome that originally came from the mother might be on the left and the paternally inherited chromosome on the right, while in another pair the opposite may be true. Then, the cell divides into two, so that only one member of the pair sorts into each of the two daughter cells. This is known as meiosis I, and at this point, there are now just 23 chromosomes per cell.

The chromosomes complete a mitotic division before entering into meiosis I. Each chromosome in the synaptic complex, therefore, has two "sister chromatid" arms that are side-by-side. (Since there is a pair of "homologous" chromosomes in each synapse, each with two sister chromatids, there are a total of four chromatids in the synapse.) The result is that the two daughter cells produced at the conclusion of meiosis I have just 23 chromosomes (a haploid quantity of chromosomes) but each chromosome is present in a duplicated form. Each daughter cell must then undergo a second event (meiosis II, which is similar to mitosis except that there are only 23 instead of 46 chromosomes). During meiosis II, the sister chromatids are pulled apart and each of the 23, now non-duplicated chromosomes with just a single chromatid per each arm, goes into two more daughter cells. The result is that there are now four daughter cells, each with a haploid quantity of nonduplicated chromosomes.

In the formation of a sperm, one diploid cell begins meiosis and four haploid spermatozoa result from it. A significant difference during oogenesis in the female is that only one haploid oocyte results. One of the daughter cells resulting from meiosis I is discarded, and one of the daughter cells resulting from meiosis II is also discarded. These discarded cells are known as "polar bodies." Another significant way that meiosis differs between the sexes is that for males, meiosis is a continuous activity that begins at puberty and continues until death. For females, there are several thousand primitive oocytes in the developing ovary of a female embryo that actually initiate meiosis I well before birth, but then arrest during embryonic development. Meiosis does not resume until after puberty, and then in only one egg at a time (with the egg that is ovulated during a particular menstrual cycle, at which point meiosis I is completed). Meiosis then again arrests, and meiosis II is not completed until just after fertilization, at which point the second polar body is ejected.

> Male meiosis produces four spermatozoa from a single germ cell precursor; female meiosis produces just one oocyte from a single germ cell precursor, discarding two polar bodies in the process.

The second responsibility of meiosis is to provide an opportunity for genetic recombination. During genetic recombination, an individual's two parental chromosome homologs actually physically break and recombine to produce a recombinant chromosome, which contains combinations of grandparental alleles that were not previously present in either parent. Recombination occurs in only two of the four chromatids present in the synapse (Fig. 2-4). So, from every meiotic event there are always two potential recombinant chromosomes (that represent reciprocal exchanges) and two non-recombinant chromosomes.

> Another difference in meiosis between women and men is that there are more recombination events (synapses) in women than in men.

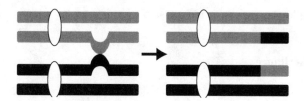

Figure 2-4   Chromosomal recombination.

MENDELIAN
INHERITANCE

·

- **Probability Review**
- **Pedigree Symbols**
- **Homozygosity and Heterozygosity**
- **Mendelian Patterns of Inheritance**
  Autosomal Dominant
    Penetrance and expressivity
      Incomplete penetrance
      Sex-dependent penetrance
      Age-dependent penetrance
    Bayes' Theorem
  Autosomal Recessive
      Hardy-Weinberg law
      Consanguinity
      Co-dominant inheritance
  Sex-linked Recessive
      Lyonization
  Unusual Forms of Inheritance
  Mitochondrial
      Imprinting
      Germline mosaicism
      Autosomal dominant nonviable

·   ·   ·   ·   ·   ·   ·   ·   ·   ·   ·   ·

PROBABILITY REVIEW

Mendelian inheritance involves three simple statistical concepts: for independent events, multiply probabilities; for mutually exclusive events, add probabilities; and, the total probability of all possible outcomes must sum to one.

The best example is a coin toss. Each time the coin is tossed, the probability of achieving heads or tail is one-half, and is independent of any prior tosses. "Chance has no memory" to the extent that, even if there had been a run of heads, the next toss is no more or less likely to be a tails than if there had been a run of tails. The likelihood of having two consecutive heads is $\frac{1}{2} \times \frac{1}{2} = \left(\frac{1}{2}\right)^2 = \frac{1}{4}$, or the probability of having three tails in a row is just $\frac{1}{2} \times \frac{1}{2} \times \frac{1}{2} = \left(\frac{1}{2}\right)^3 = \frac{1}{8}$. Note that when you flip a coin, the two possible outcomes are heads or tails; therefore, the sum of the probabilities of each outcome must add up to a total probability of one (corresponding to a certain outcome). So, for a coin tossed three times consecutively, each of the eight possible outcomes occurs with an equal probability of 1 in 8 (Fig. 3-1).

Multiply independent probabilities

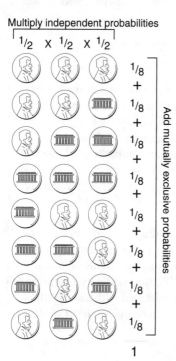

Figure 3-1   Potential outcomes of a coin toss performed three times in a row.

Let us work out a few simple genetic problems illustrating probability concepts. What is the chance that a pregnant woman will give birth to a boy? Well, that is an easy one; it is about $\frac{1}{2}$. What is the probability that she will have a girl? Same answer. So, since these are mutually exclusive probabilities, we know that the probability that she will give birth to either a boy or a girl must be one. Reassuringly, that also happens to be the sum of $\frac{1}{2}$ plus $\frac{1}{2}$.

Now let us go a step further. What is the probability that a woman will have two boys in a row? Since these are independent events we know that it must be $\frac{1}{2}$ times $\frac{1}{2}$, which equals $\frac{1}{4}$. What about two girls in a row? Same thing. How about one boy and one girl? For a family of two children, you can only have either two boys, two girls, or a boy and a girl, so the probability of a boy and a girl must equal the probability of not having two boys or two girls (since these are mutually exclusive events summing to one), and that is merely $1 - \frac{1}{4} - \frac{1}{4} = \frac{1}{2}$. But why is it twice as likely to have a boy and a girl as having two boys or two girls? That's because there are two different ways to have a boy and a girl. The boy could be born first, followed by a girl, and the chance of that sequence happening is also $\frac{1}{2} \times \frac{1}{2} = \frac{1}{4}$. Or, the girl could be born first, followed by a boy, and the chance of that sequence happening is the same. Taking those two different orders together gives a probability of 1 in 2. And everything sums to one. Let us try a trick question. Since the probability of having a boy is 1 in 2 for every child, would you agree that if one has two children, the probability of having a boy should be one? Of course not! Otherwise, every family of two children would have two boys.

PEDIGREE SYMBOLS

To simplify recording the family history, we make use of schematic symbols (Fig. 3-2). Males are square, females are round. Deceased individuals have a diagonal slash through them. Affected individuals are filled-in. Horizontal lines connecting people denote social relationships (usually solid for husband and wife, dashed when unmarried, and an interrupted line for individuals who are now divorced or otherwise estranged) and vertical lines denote descent (parent-child relationship). By custom, try to put the male in a pair on the left. Within a sibship, try to order children left to right by declining age. Diamonds are used when the sex is unspecified. Multiple individuals of a single sex can be denoted by putting a number in the middle of the square or circle. For multiple individuals of both sexes, use a diamond with a number in the middle. The notation for a fetus or pending pregnancy is typically a diamond with a "P" in the middle. Spontaneous abortion and termination of pregnancy is often denoted with a small triangle, with and without a slash, respectively. The "proband" is the individual

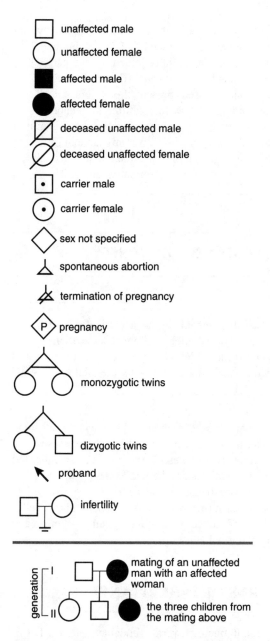

Figure 3-2   The meanings of the symbols in a pedigree.

who brought the family to attention and is denoted with a short arrow. Dizygotic (fraternal) twins usually have a horizontal line connecting them, whereas monozygotic (identical) twins are usually joined by two parallel horizontal lines. The symbols are shaded to indicate affliction with a particular disease. When more than one disease is present, the symbols may be sectored like pieces of pie, depending on how many different phenotypes one wishes to call to attention. A legend is used to define the shading and any unusual symbols or abbreviations. Sometimes, we only have information about one parent. In those cases, the inconsequential parent is usually excluded and a single vertical line is used to connect parent and child.

HOMOZYGOSITY AND HETEROZYGOSITY

Heterozygous: Having two different alleles at a particular locus, usually in reference to one normal allele and one disease allele.
Homozygous: Having two identical alleles at a particular locus, usually in reference to two normal alleles or two disease alleles.

Since an individual has two parents who each contribute one chromosome in a homologous pair to a gamete, there are two copies of each chromosome, a maternal and paternal, and therefore, two copies of every gene, one inherited from each parent. Consequently, when alleles are defined as being "diseased" or "normal," then an individual can have either identical copies of the same allele (homozygous) or different copies of each (heterozygous) for a particular gene. In reality, there are many alleles for a particular gene in a population—both many normal and, often times, several abnormal alleles.

MENDELIAN PATTERNS OF INHERITANCE

Phenotypes may be inherited through one of several mendelian patterns. Let us consider each in turn and introduce some other concepts, along with each form of inheritance:

AUTOSOMAL DOMINANT

In autosomal dominant inheritance the responsible gene is on an "autosome" (a chromosome that is not the X or Y sex chromosome and is, therefore, not sex linked). The mutation acts dominantly in that the normal allele is insufficient to compensate for the mutant allele. Heterozygotes with one copy of the disease allele and one normal allele are affected. (Homozygotes for the disease allele are generally rare. For some diseases, they are much more severely affected, and for others, there is no difference in phenotype with the heterozygous state. In general, you do not need to worry about homozygotes for the diseased allele in autosomal dominant disorders, because of their rarity.) Since one mutant allele has to overcome the effects of a normal allele simultaneously present within the cell, the molecular or cellular effect of the mutation is either "dominant negative" or "toxic gain of function," or occasionally, "haploinsufficiency" (half the level of expression from just the normal allele is not sufficient).

CHARACTERISTICS OF AUTOSOMAL DOMINANT INHERITANCE

- There is vertical transmission of the phenotype, with an affected child usually having an affected parent (except with reduced penetrance, new mutation, germline mosaicism, or anticipation).
- At conception, the chance of transmitting the phenotype from affected parent to affected child is 1 in 2.
- An unaffected individual not inheriting the phenotype has no risk of transmitting the phenotype to his or her own children (except with reduced penetrance or anticipation). In other words, there is no carrier state.
- Males and females are just as likely to transmit the phenotype, unlike the case for sex-linked recessive disorders where the phenotype is transmitted through carrier females and there is no male-to-male transmission.
- New mutations are relatively common, sometimes accounting for up to half or more of all patients, and depends on the fitness of the syndrome.

EXAMPLE: MARFAN SYNDROME

Marfan syndrome is a hereditary disease characterized by involvement of three organ systems, the skeleton, eyes, and cardiovascular system. Skeletal manifestations are comprised of disproportionately long extremities (dolichostenomelia), long fingers and toes (arachnodactyly), "pigeon" or "funnel" sternal chest deformity (pectus carinatum or pectus excavatum, respectively), and lateral curvature of the spine (scoliosis). The ophthalmologic abnormalities consist of near-sightedness (myopia) and lens dislocation (ectopia lentis). The major cardiovascular abnormality is a risk for aortic aneurysm and dissection. Mitral valve prolapse may also be present. Treatment with beta-blockers slows progressive dilatation of the aortic root and risk for aneurysm of the ascending aorta. Mutations in the fibrillin gene on chromosome 15 have been identified as the molecular genetic cause of Marfan syndrome.

In the pedigree shown in Figure 3-3, every affected individual has a 1 in 2 probability of transmitting Marfan syndrome to each of his or her offspring. Thus, the chance that the fetus will inherit Marfan syndrome from his or her affected mother is 1 in 2.

One useful tool for illustrating mendelian inheritance is the Punnett square (Fig. 3-4). Here, it can be seen that the affected mother's genotype is A/a, where "a" represents the mutant allele for the gene causing Marfan syndrome and "A" represents a "normal" or non-disease causing allele. We put the maternal genotype horizontally on top of the Punnett square and note that during maternal meiosis, there is an equal (and hence, 1 in 2) probability of transmitting either the a or A allele to the oocyte. The unaffected father's genotype is placed vertically on the side of the Punnett square and is denoted as A/A, since it is inferred that he has two normal alleles of the fibrillin gene causing Marfan syndrome. Again, during paternal meiosis, the chance of sending either normal allele to the spermatozoa is equal and is 1 in 2. Since paternal and maternal meiosis are independent events, we just multiply the individual probabilities to determine the probability that both will happen. From the Punnett square, then, we can see that there are four possible outcomes, each with probability of $\frac{1}{2} \times \frac{1}{2} = \frac{1}{4}$. (Reassuringly, the probabilities for all of the possible outcomes sums to one, since we know that one of these must actually happen.) Two of the outcomes result in a conception who

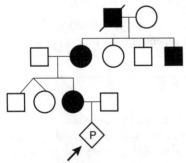

What is the probability that this
pending pregnancy will be affected?   **Figure 3-3   Example: Marfan syndrome.**

maternal
A
a
paternal
A
A
AA
Aa
AA
Aa
1/2 unaffected
1/2 affected

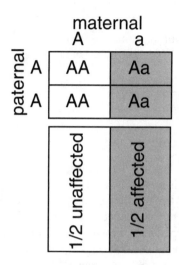

Figure 3-4 Punnett square for autosomal dominant inheritance.

inherits Marfan syndrome (producing the genotype A/a), while two of the outcomes yield a conception who does not inherit Marfan syndrome (A/A). The probability that the conception will have inherited Marfan syndrome is, therefore, the total of the squares in the diagram that yield genotype a/A (two) divided by the total number of possible outcomes (four), and that is $\frac{1}{2}$. The probability that the conception will not have inherited Marfan syndrome is similarly the total of the squares in the diagram that produce the genotype A/A, and that also occurs in two squares out of four $\left(\text{or } \frac{1}{2}\right)$. Again, the sum of these mutually exclusive events is one. Some people prefer to draw out a "branching diagram," which is also illustrated in Figure 3-5, as an alternative method for solving the problem.

Penetrance and expressivity

It is important to realize that the phenotype may not appear in all individuals or, if it is present, may not be the same between different individuals. The former concept refers to "penetrance," and the latter relates to "expressivity."

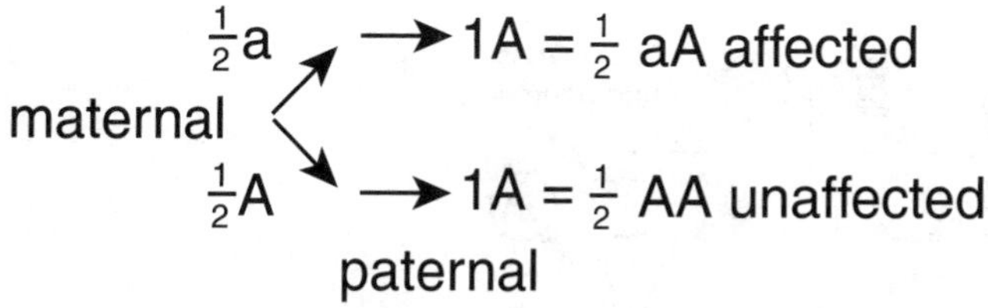

1/2 a
maternal
1/2 A
1A = 1/2 aA affected
1A = 1/2 AA unaffected
paternal

Figure 3-5 Branching diagrams for autosomal dominant inheritance.

> **Penetrance:** Probability that a gene will have any phenotypic expression at all. In contrast to expressivity, severity is not taken into account.

Incomplete penetrance

EXAMPLE: FACTOR V LEIDEN DEFICIENCY

Factor V is a component of the blood clotting cascade. The Leiden mutation (named after the city in the Netherlands where it was discovered) consists of a particular amino acid substitution that impairs the function of factor V. Heterozygotes for the factor V Leiden allele have a hypercoagulable state that leads to a risk for developing venous blood clots (deep venous thrombosis, or DVTs) in the extremities. DVTs are at risk to dislodge and travel to the lungs (pulmonary embolus, or PEs), which can lead to significant hypoxemic shunting of blood flow through the lungs and often, death. It is now known that factor V Leiden deficiency is one of the major risk factors for developing venous thrombosis. As many as 40% of Caucasian individuals presenting with a DVT may be factor V Leiden heterozygotes. Because the factor V Leiden allele confers hypercoagulability in the heterozygous state, it is inherited in an autosomal dominant fashion. The clinical phenotype, venous thrombosis, will manifest over the lifetime of only about 50% of heterozygotes, however. We call this phenomenon, then, incomplete penetrance, in that not everyone who inherits the mutation will have clinical manifestations of the disease (Fig. 3-6). Can you think of some reasons for incomplete penetrance? You might know some other risk factors for DVTs and PEs. These other risk factors include recent sedentary activity (such as a long airline or automobile trip or a postoperative patient confined to bed), pregnancy, the presence of a central venous catheter, oral contraceptive use, men with well developed upper limb musculature, and other genetic factors contributing to hypercoagulability. Thus, it is a combination of other genes and environmental factors, which differs between individuals, that accounts for incomplete penetrance.

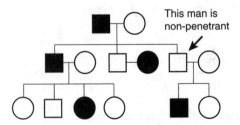

Figure 3-6 Example: Factor V Leiden deficiency.

Sex-dependent penetrance

EXAMPLE: BRCA2 FAMILIAL BREAST CANCER

BRCA2 is one gene responsible for familial breast cancer. (We will discuss this topic in greater detail in the chapter on cancer genetics.) Men who belong to a BRCA2 breast cancer family can also develop breast cancer, albeit somewhat infrequently (Fig. 3-7). With BRCA2 mutations, the penetrance for breast cancer is greatly reduced in males, an example of sex-dependent penetrance. The reasons for this seem obvious: males have less breast tissue, and the breast tissue that is present is not hormonally stimulated.

Age-dependent penetrance

EXAMPLE: HUNTINGTON'S DISEASE

Huntington's disease is an autosomal dominant neurodegenerative disease characterized by a frank dance-like movement disorder known as chorea. Anatomically, there is focal degeneration of the caudate nucleus in the brain. There is no effective treatment other than symptomatic control of chorea with antidopaminergic agents. Mutations in the gene, huntingtin, are responsible for the disease. The mutations are always expansions of polyglutamine encoding CAG trinucleotide repeat tracts (more on this later). The disease demonstrates age-dependent penetrance, in that, unlike some illnesses where the phenotype is present at birth, phenotypic manifestations, and hence diagnosis, rarely occur before adulthood. In the pedigree shown in Figure 3-8, we wish to calculate the probability that a woman who is presently 30 years old inherited Huntington's disease from her affected father, knowing that at this age, she is asymptomatic. From published epidemiologic studies, we have available data correlating the age of onset of symptoms and signs of Huntington's disease in individuals heterozygous for mutations in huntingtin. How do we go about applying this data toward the risk calculation posed in this example pedigree? To do so, we need to digress into another aspect of probability, known as Bayes' theorem.

Bayes' theorem

The Reverend Thomas Bayes was an eighteenth century English mathematician whose famous theorem was published only after his death. Bayes' theorem offers

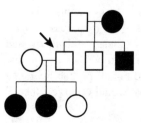

Figure 3-7   Example: BRCA2 familial breast cancer.
Although men can get breast cancer, penetrance is much lower than in woman who inherit BRCA2 mutations.

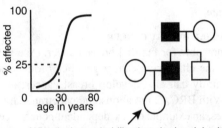

What is the probability that she has inherited a
huntingtin mutation given that she's unaffected at 30?

Figure 3-8   Example: Huntington's disease.

a formal means to change probability estimates to take into account new information. The process involves changing a "prior probability" based on new data ("conditional probability") to calculate a "posterior probability."

There are two frequent applications of Bayes' theorem in medical genetics. One is when calculating the probability that someone inherited an autosomal dominant disease demonstrating age-dependent penetrance when they are at a given age and remain unaffected (our present example). Another application is calculating the probability that someone is a carrier of a sex-linked or autosomal recessive disease after they have already had some number of unaffected children (an example we will shortly come to).

Much as you learned to do long division, most people have found it useful to use either one of two different algorithms when employing Bayes' theorem, and we will work the problem here using these two common methods.

We will first work it out using a table-based method, in which we have two columns with three rows each (Fig. 3-9). In this example, we must first calculate the so-called prior probability that she either inherited or did not inherit the gene for Huntington's disease. Because this is an autosomal dominant disease where heterozygotes are affected, we can easily infer that her father was a heterozygote for huntingtin mutations and that, at conception, the risk that she would inherit the mutant huntingtin allele from her father was simply $\frac{1}{2}$. And, of course, the risk that she did not inherit the mutant huntingtin allele was also $\frac{1}{2}$ (and, reassuringly, they sum to 1). So, we start by making two columns, one labeled "did inherit" and the other labeled "did not inherit." The entry for our first row (the prior probability) is $\frac{1}{2}$ in each column. Next, we calculate the "conditional" probability in the second row of this table. This is the probability that we would observe either of

probability	did inherit	did not inherit
prior	$\frac{1}{2}$	$\frac{1}{2}$
conditional	$\frac{3}{4}$	1
joint	$\frac{1}{2} \times \frac{3}{4} = \frac{3}{8}$	$\frac{1}{2} \times 1 = \frac{1}{2}$
posterior probability of inheriting knowing she is asymptomatic at age 30	$\dfrac{\frac{3}{8}}{\frac{3}{8}+\frac{1}{2}} = \frac{3}{7} \approx 43\%$	

Figure 3-9   Application of Bayes' theorem using the table approach.

the situations in the column headings given the information that we now have (that she is unaffected at age 30). Let us do the right column first, since that is the easier situation. What we are after for this entry in the table is the probability that she would be clinically unaffected at age 30, if she did not inherit the gene for Huntington's disease. This is easy, and the answer is 1. (If she didn't inherit the mutant allele then she has no chance of having Huntington's disease regardless of her age.) Now let us do the entry for the left column in this second row. Here, we ask the question of what is the probability that she would be clinically unaffected at age 30 if she were to have inherited the gene for Huntington's disease. Here is where we make use of the data for age-dependent penetrance. We see that by age 30, only about 25% of huntingtin mutation heterozygotes will have clinical manifestations of Huntington's disease. So, 75% ($\frac{3}{4}$) of individuals who have inherited huntingtin mutations will remain clinically unaffected by the time they reach this age. We therefore record $\frac{3}{4}$ for this entry in the table. (Note that the conditional probabilities of the second row are not mutually exclusive outcomes, since we are supposing two completely different scenarios. Unlike the case for the first row of prior probabilities, we, therefore, do not expect that these two probabilities should sum to one, and they do not.) The third row is known as the joint probability. This is just the product of the two entries for each column in the previous two rows. The joint probability in the left column is just $\frac{1}{2} \times \frac{3}{4} = \frac{3}{8}$, and the joint probability in the right column is just $\frac{1}{2} \times 1 = \frac{1}{2}$. To finish up, we must calculate the posterior probability. What we are after is the probability that the hypothetical situation in the first column is true (that she inherited the huntingtin mutation but remains clinically unaffected at age 30). You might be tempted to just take the joint probability for this situation, but you cannot do that. The reason is that the joint probabilities that we have calculated in the third row do not sum to one. In constructing this table, we actually threw out one possible scenario. We threw out the possibility that if she did inherit the gene, that she would be affected. We threw it away because we know her to be clinically unaffected. In other words, since we have discarded one of the mutually exclusive probabilities, we have to correct for the only two possible outcomes that are made tenable by the facts of this case. Making this correction is simple. We set up a fraction. The numerator is simply the joint probability we are interested in, that she inherited the mutation from her father but is clinically unaffected at age 30 because of age-dependent penetrance, and this is $\frac{3}{8}$. The denominator is the sum of the only two possible outcomes that the facts allow. She either inherited the mutation from her father but remains clinically unaffected at age 30, or she did not inherit the mutation from her father and is necessarily, clinically unaffected. The denominator is, therefore, $\frac{3}{8}$ plus $\frac{1}{2}$. In summary, to calculate the posterior probability from the information in the table, we set up a fraction in which the numerator contains the joint probability for the situation we are interested in, and the denominator contains the sum of the joint probabilities from the two columns of the table. We solve the problem arithmetically and find that the answer is 3/7 (43%). Therefore, the risk that she inherited the Huntington's disease gene and will one day develop the disease, is 43%. Note that the risk has gone down from her $\frac{1}{2}$ risk present at conception, and that the longer she lives without developing symptoms, the less this risk will become. For example, if she continues to remain asymptomatic by age 45, where the age-dependent penetrance for Huntington's disease is 50%, then the probability that she actually inherited the mutant allele from her father will be $\frac{1}{3}$. (You should work this out yourself to make sure you understand how to do these sorts of problems. Hint, just substitute $\frac{1}{2}$ in the second row of the left column of the table and take it from there.) Should she remain asymptomatic by about age 85, where penetrance reaches 100%, then we can completely exclude the possibility that she inherited the mutation for Huntington's disease.

Now let us work it out a different way, using a branching diagram (Fig. 3-10). (In our experience, most people have a preference for one of the two illustrated methods, but the population of medical students is probably equally divided on which approach is preferable.) We will start by saying that at conception the patient in this example has a 1 in 2 probability of inheriting the mutant allele causing Huntington's disease and has a 1 in 2 probability of not inheriting the mutant gene. This is shown by alternate directions on the diagram. For the bottom arrow, that she did not inherit the mutant gene, the probability that she will be clinically unaffected at age 30 is just one. (And, of course, the probability that she will be affected if she did not inherit it is zero, an outcome we can ignore.) For the top row, there are two different possibilities, denoted by two more arrows branching off into different directions. With respect to this second set of arrows, for the top arrow, there is a 1 in 4 probability that she will manifest symptoms at age 30 if she inherited the mutant gene. For the bottom arrow, there is a 3 in 4 chance that she will be clinically unaffected at age 30 if she inherited

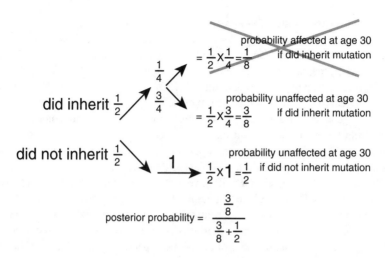

Figure 3-10   Branching diagram approach to Bayes' theorem.

the mutant gene. We now have three possible outcomes, the joint probability for which is merely the product of all the preceding events. Thus, from top to bottom, the probability that she inherited the mutation and is clinically affected is $\frac{1}{2}$ $\times \frac{1}{4} = \frac{1}{8}$; the probability that she inherited the mutation and is clinically unaffected is $\frac{1}{2} \times \frac{3}{4} = \frac{3}{8}$; and, the probability that she did not inherit the mutation and is clinically unaffected is $\frac{1}{2} \times 1 = \frac{1}{2}$. (Reassuringly, the sum of all three mutually exclusive outcomes is, indeed, 1.) But, we know that she is clinically unaffected at age 30, so we can cross off the first of the possibilities. Now, we must calculate the posterior probability, just as we did before using the table method. Since we excluded one of the possible outcomes, and the sum of the two tenable outcomes is no longer one, we must "normalize" this. So, just as before, the denominator in the fraction expressing posterior probability is just the sum of the only two possible outcomes that are left, $\frac{1}{2} + \frac{3}{4}$. The numerator is the outcome we are after, that she inherited the mutation but did not develop disease, and this is $\frac{3}{4}$. Again, we arithmetically solve this as before.

Expressivity

> **Expressivity:** The degree of expression of the phenotype. Unlike penetrance, expressivity takes into account varying breadth and/or severity of the clinical features of a disease. The term is most often used in the context of variable expressivity.

EXAMPLE: WAARDENBURG SYNDROME

Each member of the family (Fig. 3-11) has different manifestations of the syndrome. One has deafness, another has pigmentary changes, the third has both deafness and pigmentary changes. Waardenburg syndrome is an autosomal dominant disorder caused by mutations in the PAX3 gene on chromosome 2. There is a cellular defect in the migration of neural crest cells during embryogenesis, with a resultant phenotype affecting aspects of pigmentation (the melanosomes being derived from the neural crest) and nervous system development. There is often present, as well, a characteristic facial appearance (facies). It is easy to envision one source for variable expressivity of Waardenburg syndrome between affected individuals. Simply, not everyone will have the same mutation. Individuals from different families will have different mutant alleles. (This is known as allelic heterogeneity, a topic to which we shall return later.) In the particular case of Waardenburg syndrome and many other inherited diseases, however, even individuals within the same family, who would of course be expected to have the exact same mutant allele, will demonstrate variable expressivity, with a differing intensity and spectrum of disease. Can you think of some explanations? The answers are basically the same as those accounting for incomplete penetrance: somewhat weaker effects of so-called "modifying" genes (what is also referred to as the "genetic background" of an individual) and differing environmental exposures between the individuals. For example, deafness could be influenced by occupational exposure to noise.

AUTOSOMAL RECESSIVE

Recessive implies that both alleles must be defective. It is frequently due to a loss of function, molecularly resulting from inactivation of the gene. Genes can be inactivated through a variety of different particular types of mutations, but deletions are perhaps the most common way that a recessively acting allele occurs. Affected individuals are homozygous for the disease allele as are the children of parents who are both unaffected heterozygous carriers of the disease allele.

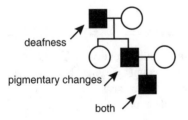

deafness ↗

pigmentary changes ↗

both ↗

Figure 3-11   Example: Waardenburg syndrome.
Each member of this family has different manifestations of the syndrome.

CHARACTERISTICS OF AUTOSOMAL RECESSIVE INHERITANCE

- If it appears in more than one family member, typically it is seen only within a sibship, not in other generations.
- The likelihood that two carrier parents will yield an affected conception is 25%.
- More common with consanguinity, especially for rare diseases.
- Usually, males and females are equally likely to be affected.
- New mutation is almost never a consideration.

EXAMPLE: CYSTIC FIBROSIS

Cystic fibrosis (CF) is among the most common autosomal recessive diseases in the Caucasian population. It results from mutations in CFTR, a transmembrane chloride ion channel. Defects in chloride electrolyte metabolism were appreciated long before the cloning of the gene, and the "gold standard" for diagnosis was, and still is, a chloride sweat test, which measures the chloride ion concentration in a small patch of skin induced to sweat by treatment with a parasympathomimetic agent. The defect in the chloride channel leads to a viscous mucous production which, in turn, leads to pathology in primarily three organ systems. Most serious are the pulmonary complications. The bronchioles become progressively dilated, inelastic, and mucous impacted (bronchiectasis), and the lungs become recurrently, then chronically, infected with *Pseudomonas* and other bacterial species. Eventually, the bacteria become resistant to most or all antibiotics in almost all patients. The terminal event is often intractable pneumonia and severe hemoptysis (coughing up of blood that has flowed into the lungs). The only definitive treatment is lung transplant. Pancreatic exocrine insufficiency is also frequently seen in CF patients, resulting in malabsorption. Azoospermia with male infertility is apparent, although, except for the encumbrances of a chronic disease, women with CF can be fertile. There is good "genotype-phenotype" correlation in CF, in that the particular combination of mutant alleles tends to determine both the severity and spectrum of the disease. Seventy percent of the mutant alleles in the Caucasian population are the "ΔF508," corresponding to a three nucleotide in-frame deletion that inactivates chloride ion channel activity by causing a loss of a critically important phenylalanine at amino acid position 508 of the CFTR protein. The classic ΔF508 homozygote has severe lung disease as well as pancreatic exocrine deficiency.

In the pedigree shown in Figure 3-12, we wish to know what is the probability that the fetus in the pending pregnancy inherited CF, given that this couple has already had two children affected with CF. Since CF is an autosomal

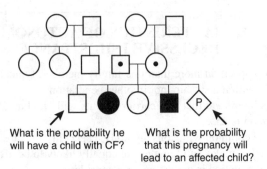

What is the probability he   What is the probability
will have a child with CF?   that this pregnancy will
                                 lead to an affected child?

Figure 3-12   Example: Cystic fibrosis.

recessive disease, we can infer that both parents are heterozygote carriers of CF mutations. They, thus, have one normal allele for CFTR and one disease allele. We put a dot in the middle of their pedigree symbols to denote the fact that they are inferred to be obligate heterozygotes. We can set up a Punnett square (Fig. 3-13). In this case, we put the carrier mother horizontally on the top and denote her genotype as A/a, where A corresponds to the normal allele and a represents the mutant allele. We place the father vertically on the left with the same A/a genotype. Since there is a 1 in 2 probability of segregating either the a or A allele into the sperm or egg during meiosis in the father or mother, respectively, we can see that there are four possible outcomes, each with equal probability of $\frac{1}{4}$. Since there are two different ways to produce a carrier state, the probability that the fetus will be a carrier is $\frac{1}{4} + \frac{1}{4} = \frac{1}{2}$. It should be clear that the probability that the fetus will have genotype a/a and inherit CF is 1 in 4, while the probability that the fetus will be homozgyous for two normal alleles A/A is also 1 in 4. Reassuringly, the sum of these mutually exclusive and complete outcomes is 1. We can also work this out using a branching diagram (Fig. 3-14).

Now let us try a tricky question. What is the probability that the unaffected brother will be a carrier? You might be tempted to say 1 in 2, but that is an incor-

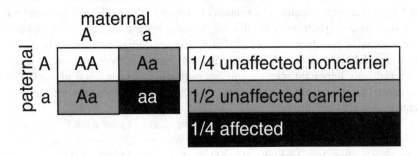

Figure 3-13   Punnett square for autosomal recessive inheritance.

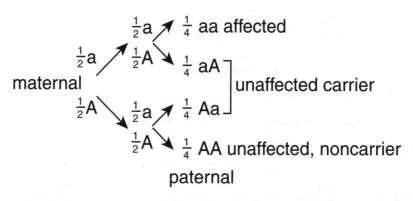

Figure 3-14   Branching diagram for autosomal recessive inheritance.

rect answer. We know that he does not have CF (the black smaller square), so we can eliminate this from the four possible outcomes and cross this off of our Punnett square. This leaves only three possible outcomes in the Punnett square, and we must reset these outcomes so that they sum to 1. Since we know that they all originally had equal probabilities, each of the three remaining small squares in our Punnett square should now have a probability of 1 in 3. Thus, the probability that he is a carrier (emphasizing that we know him to be unaffected) is 2 in 3.

Hardy-Weinberg law

The Hardy-Weinberg law is a formalization of the concept that the frequency of alleles in a large population will be constant from one generation to the next, provided that mating is random (the genotype does not influence mate selection) and that the genotype has no selective effect on success at producing offspring (Fig. 3-15), two assumptions that are, usually, correct.

> A practical implication of the Hardy-Weinberg law is that we can calculate the probability that someone is a carrier of a recessive gene solely on the basis of the prevalence of the disease in the population.

Let us refer back to the example CF pedigree and ask what is the probability that the brother will have a child with CF. We previously figured out that he has a 2 in 3 chance of being a carrier. We next need to calculate the probability that his mate will be a carrier of CF. We can do this from only knowing the prevalence of the disease in the population. (Prevalence is the total number of individuals in a population with the disease divided by the total population.) The prevalence of CF in the Caucasian population at birth is about 1/2000. Since everyone

p = frequency of one allele (here M)
q = frequency of other allele(s), by convention the less common (here N)

thus, the 3 genotypes are . . .
(M/M) p^2 = frequency of noncarriers

(M /N) pq ⎤
(N/ M) qp ⎦ $2pq$ = frequency of heterozygote carriers

(N/N) q^2 = frequency of homozygous affecteds

Figure 3-15   Hardy-Weinberg law.

with CF must have the homozgyous mutant genotype (N/N), we know that $q^2 = 1/2000$. Thus, q, the frequency of the mutant alleles in the population, equals the square root of 1/2000, which is about 0.022. We can solve for p explicitly since we know that $p + q = 1$, but we don't really need to do this for these kinds of calculations.

> It turns out that since q is usually so small, p is usually so close to one that we can just approximate $p = 1$ when using the Hardy-Weinberg equation.

The frequency of heterozygote carriers in the population is thus just $2pq$, which is approximately equal to $2q$, which is 0.044. So about 4.4% of the Caucasian population are CF carriers, corresponding to about 1 of every 23 Caucasian people. (Note that even for a somewhat rare autosomal recessive disease like CF, heterozygote carriers are pretty common, because $2pq >> q^2$.) Thus, to calculate the probability that the brother in the above pedigree will have a child with CF, his chance of being a carrier $\left(\frac{2}{3}\right)$ is multiplied times the chance that, if he were a carrier, he would transmit the mutant allele during the meiosis producing his sperm $\left(\frac{1}{2}\right)$, times the chance that his mate randomly selected from the Caucasian population would be also be a carrier (1/23), times the chance that—should she be a carrier—that she would transmit the mutant allele during the meiosis producing her egg $\left(\frac{1}{2}\right)$. And the answer is $\frac{2}{3} \times \frac{1}{2} \times 1/23 \times \frac{1}{2} = 0.008$, or about 0.8%.

EXAMPLE: HEMOCHROMATOSIS
It should be emphasized that incomplete penetrance and variable expressivity both occur with autosomal recessive disease (or sex-linked recessive inheritance, which we will discuss shortly), just as is the case with autosomal dominant inheritance. A good example of an autosomal recessive disease that demonstrates every aspect of incomplete penetrance and variable expressivity is hemochromatosis. Hemochromatosis, or "iron overload syndrome," is considered to be among the most common recessive diseases in the Caucasian population. It

results from mutations in a component of the human leukocyte antigen (HLA) complex, known as HLA-H, which is somehow involved in the regulation of iron metabolism. A single allele resulting in a missense amino acid substitution accounts for about 88% of all mutant alleles in the Caucasian population. The disease manifests clinically with cirrhosis and consequent risk for hepatocellular carcinoma, a unique arthritis, bronzing of the skin, cardiomyopathy, diabetes mellitus, and, in males, testicular atrophy. It is rather simply treated, if diagnosed early enough, with periodic phlebotomy, since the red blood cell mass represents the major form of storage of iron in the body. It used to be definitively diagnosed through liver biopsy and corroborating laboratory studies, including increased levels of serum ferritin and transferrin. Recently, DNA diagnostic studies using PCR have become the gold standard. Not everyone who is homozygous for the most common mutant allele will develop symptoms of hemochromatosis. Thus, this disease demonstrates incomplete penetrance. The reasons for this are that not everyone is exposed to the same environmental and genetic factors. The environmental factors would include dietary iron intake. Genetic factors modifying hemochromatosis risk still remain largely unknown, however. Furthermore, this disease demonstrates age-dependent penetrance. A homozygote is much more likely to have clinical hemochromatosis with advancing age, merely because it takes some time for the toxic accumulation of iron in organs. The disease also demonstrates sex-dependent penetrance. Since women menstruate and have an average lower red blood cell mass, their total body iron stores tend to be less than those of males, and they are less likely to develop organ toxicity. Furthermore, the disease demonstrates variable expressivity, in that not everyone who has hemochromatosis will have exactly the same range of clinical severity or same pattern of organ system involvement. For example, obese individuals and those with other hereditary risk for diabetes mellitus might be more likely to develop this complication of the disease. Individuals who also abuse ethanol may be more likely to develop cirrhosis.

Consanguinity

"Consanguinity" refers to relationship by descent from a common ancestor (also known as inbreeding). Consanguinity is a concern in autosomal recessive disease because, if it is a rare disease (due to an infrequent allele), the disease will occur more commonly in individuals whose parents are related. Consanguinity is noted on a pedigree by two horizontal lines between the male and female partner.

Always consider the possibility of consanguinity when approaching a patient with an autosomal recessive disease, especially when the disease is rare.

EXAMPLE: PHENYLKETONURIA

In the example illustrated in Figure 3-16, we can see how there is an increased probability of a recessive disease, phenylketonuria (PKU), occurring in a pregnancy resulting from a consanguineous mating. PKU most commonly results from deficiency of phenylalanine hydroxylase involved in the metabolism of the amino acid phenylalanine. This leads to the accumulation of neurotoxic levels of phenylalanine. Clinical manifestations include mental retardation, seizure disorder, a "mousy" odor, and hypopigmentation of skin and hair. Children who inherit the metabolic defect, but who avoid dietary exposure to high concentrations of phenylalanine, however, are essentially normal. PKU screening at birth has, therefore, become routine. It is important to ask about the possibility of consanguinity when taking a family history, especially when considering the possibility of an autosomal recessive disease. The diagnosis of a rare disease in an ethnically isolated or otherwise consanguineous pedigree should make one think about the possibility of autosomal recessive inheritance.

Co-dominant inheritance

Co-dominant inheritance works like autosomal recessive inheritance, except that in this case, each allele is capable of producing an additive effect.

EXAMPLE: HLA

The best example of this is the human leukocyte antigen complex (HLA). The HLA is a cluster of genes located on the short arm of chromosome 6 and governs immune reactions. HLA compatibility is one of the chief factors in bone marrow or solid organ transplant rejection. The most well characterized HLA components are the class I antigens, A, B, C. For each of the HLA genes there are a great num-

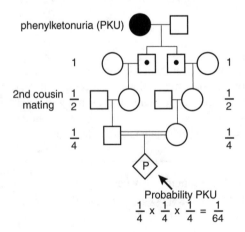

Figure 3-16   Example: Consanguinity.
Relationship by descent from a common ancestor. Seen more commonly with autosomal recessive inheritance.

ber of alleles, perhaps 50 or more, present in the population. In general, the different HLA genes are closely enough spaced, such that recombination events are infrequently observed in any given individual or family. Even without recombination, it is easy to see that with so many different HLA genes, and so many alleles for each gene, there are a great number of HLA haplotypes (or just types) in the population. (We use the term "haplotype" to describe the particular allele combinations present in closely spaced genes for a particular individual, more on this later.) However, when considering the opportunities for recombination across many generations and many individuals, recombination events are frequent enough that almost any combination of alleles for a particular HLA haplotype can be shuffled with almost any other HLA haplotype. The result is that there is an extremely large number of different HLA types present in a population, and this is one of the factors that so clinically complicates bone marrow and solid organ transplantation.

Let us look at a particular case. Bone marrow transplantation is commonly used in the treatment of leukemia, but works best when the HLA types are closely matched. This means that both the donor and recipient should have the exact same alleles for each of the markers A, B, C encoded by adjacent genes in the HLA complex. Who would be the most likely person to match a leukemic patient? Not someone drawn from random in the general population; the probability of a match is extremely low given the vast number of potential HLA types represented in the population. Not a parent, because only one allele for each locus would be inherited from a single parent, and it would be extremely unlikely for both parents to be fortuitously HLA identical. Except when there is an monozygotic twin, the best chance for a match comes from an ordinary sibling.

What is the probability that if a patient has just a single sibling that the two will be HLA matched? The problem is really rather simple. Since the HLA genes are so closely spaced and recombination is generally rare, the whole HLA locus is usually inherited together. Drawing out a Punnett square where the mother's HLA haplotype is represented as 1 and 2 and the dissimilar father's as 3 and 4 (Fig. 3-17), it is clear that there are four different haplotypes possible, and that the probability that a patient will find a match with one sibling is about $\frac{1}{4}$.

Figure 3-17 **Punnett square for inheritance of HLA types.**

> The probability that each sibling of a particular individual will be HLA matched is 1 in 4 (actually somewhat less when recombination is considered).

Now, suppose that the patient has not one sibling, but four. What is the probability for finding a match? Easy, right. . .it should be $4 \times \frac{1}{4} = 1$? Wrong, it is not so simple. (Remember, flipping a coin twice does not guarantee that you will get at least one heads.) A better way to think about the problem is what is the probability that a given sibling will NOT be an HLA match. This is just $1 - \frac{1}{4} = \frac{3}{4}$. So, the probability of being unfortunate enough to not have a match, and having four chances of doing so, is $\frac{3}{4} \times \frac{3}{4} \times \frac{3}{4} \times \frac{3}{4} = \left(\frac{3}{4}\right)^4 = 32\%$. The probability of having a match is just 1 minus this result and is 68%.

Now consider the effects of recombination in the HLA locus. Suppose that a child has leukemia and his HLA type reveals that at HLA-A, he has two alleles, A2 and A9, and at HLA-B, he has two alleles, B16 and B13 (thus, he is A2, A9; B16, B13). (We will ignore HLA-C just to make it a bit simpler.) His father is A2, A1; B7, B16 and his mother is A28, A9; B15, B13. One brother and one sister are each A2, A9; B7, B13. The other brother and sister are also matched and are each A28, A1; B15, B16. Unfortunately, then, it appears that there is no HLA match in the family for this patient. The patient's parents announce that they will attempt to have another child and will keep having more until they get a match to serve as a donor for their ill child. This really happened and was widely reported in the media, but how likely is this strategy to succeed? Well, in our hypothetical example, it is not very likely. As can be seen when the haplotypes are drawn out (Fig. 3-18), in all the other children in the family the A and B alle-

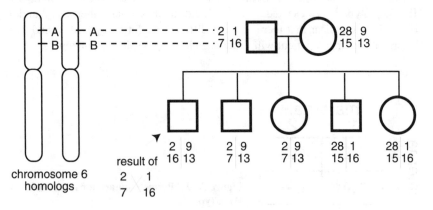

Figure 3-18   Example: HLA inheritance.

les remain on the same chromosome throughout meiotic segregation, but in the patient, there is a paternal recombination event between the A and B loci. The chance of meiotic recombination again occurring between the father's A and B loci is less than about 1% (given that the HLA-A and HLA-B loci are so close together), and, combined with the only 1 in 4 chance of inheriting the right combination of alleles, the likelihood that the next child will be a matched HLA donor for this patient is just 1 in 400. About that case where this really happened? One can only conclude that the little girl with leukemia was not a recombinant and that the family got lucky and achieved a match, in spite of the only 1 in 4 chance of success.

SEX-LINKED RECESSIVE

Sex-linked recessive inheritance (also known as X-linked recessive inheritance) occurs when the gene is on the X chromosome and acts recessively. Since females have two copies of the X chromosome, in order to be affected, both copies must be defective. This is much less likely than in the situation for males, in which there is only a single X chromosome and a non-compensatory region of the Y chromosome. Males are, therefore, considered "hemizygous" for the X chromosome. Males inherit their single X chromosome from their mother, so sex-linked recessive disease follows a maternally inherited distribution pattern in the family.

CHARACTERISTICS OF SEX-LINKED RECESSIVE INHERITANCE

- Males are more commonly affected than females.
- The gene responsible is transmitted from an affected man through his daughters, who are seldom affected. Each daughter is an obligatory heterozygous carrier. Each of the carrier daughter's sons has a 50% chance of inheriting it.
- No male-to-male transmission occurs.
- The affected males in a pedigree are usually related through females.
- Heterozygous female carriers are usually unaffected, but infrequently may demonstrate variable severity of the phenotype.

EXAMPLE: HEMOPHILIA A

Hemophilia A is among the most common of sex-linked recessive diseases. It results from a deficiency of factor VIII, a component of the blood clotting cascade. Most of the bleeding is into the joint space or into the gut. Males who have a factor VIII mutation are affected because they are hemizygous for the gene, having only one copy of the X chromosome where the gene resides. Females who have a factor VIII mutation are usually unaffected. Although they may have reduced levels of factor VIII activity (resulting from the phenomenon of X-chromosome inactivation, described as follows), this is usually enough to prevent clinical symptoms.

What is the probability that the fetus in the pending pregnancy shown in Figure 3-19 will have inherited hemophilia A? We can assume that the pregnant mother is a carrier. She has already had one affected son and there is an extensive history of hemophilia A in males in the family. (As you will see later, if there was only this one affected son, we could not exclude the possibility that he was a new mutation and that the disease is not inherited in this family.) Since the mother is a carrier, she has one normal factor VIII allele and one mutant factor VIII allele. The probability that she will transmit the mutant allele during oogenesis is, therefore, 1 in 2. The probability that the fetus will have the mutant factor VIII allele is also 1 in 2. In this case, the sex of the fetus is important. If the fetus inherits an X chromosome from the father and is female, she will probably not be affected with hemophilia A (although there are some exceptions that we will discuss). So, we need really only be concerned with the possibility that the fetus inherits a Y chromosome from the father and is a male—an event with probability of 1 in 2. The product of these two independent events, the $\frac{1}{2}$ probability that the mother will contribute her mutant factor VIII allele to the egg and the $\frac{1}{2}$ probability that the father will contribute a Y and make the conceptus a male, is $\frac{1}{4}$, and this is the probability that the fetus will be a male inheriting hemophilia A. Again, one can draw out a Punnett square (Fig. 3-20) or a branching diagram (Fig. 3-21), but we should start to be able to see these things by now without the aid of such didactic tools.

Now try a more difficult problem that requires the use of Bayes' theorem. We will determine the probability that the woman indicated in the pedigree is actually a carrier of hemophilia A after giving birth to three unaffected children.

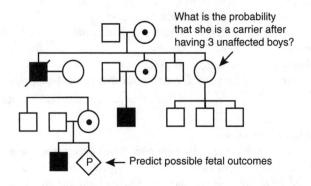

Figure 3-19   Example: Hemophilia A.

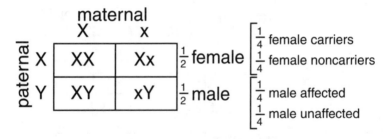

Figure 3-20   Punnett square for sex-linked recessive inheritance.

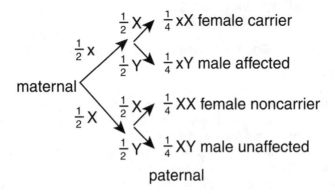

Figure 3-21   Branching diagram for sex-linked recessive inheritance.

Again, we will work this out using each of the two methods. For the table method (Fig. 3-22), we construct two columns, that she either is a carrier (on the left) or that she is not a carrier (on the right). Note that her mother appears to be a carrier, since her brother is affected. The probability that the indicated woman inherited a factor VIII mutation at birth is, thus, 1 in 2. The prior probability of her being either a carrier or a noncarrier is 1 in 2, so we enter $\frac{1}{2}$ in both columns of the first row of the table. Next, we calculate the conditional probability in the second row. Let us do the right column first, since that is the easy one. What we want to know is the probability that we would observe her to have had three unaffected sons if she were not a carrier. This is easy; the answer here is one. (If she were not a carrier, then she is not going to have affected boys.) Now, for the entry in the left column, we need to ask what is the probability that she would have three unaffected boys if she were a carrier. Well, every time she has a boy, there is a 1 in 2 probability that the boy will inherit her factor VIII mutant allele. So, the probability of having three unaffected boys, if she were a carrier, is $\frac{1}{2} \times \frac{1}{2} \times \frac{1}{2} = \left(\frac{1}{2}\right)^3 = \frac{1}{8}$, and this is what we enter in the table. (This can get a bit tricky here. We do not have to consider the probability of having boys or girls. What we do know is that she had three boys. Each of the boys is unaffected. So, perhaps a better way

probability	carrier	noncarrier
prior	$\frac{1}{2}$	$\frac{1}{2}$
conditional	$(\frac{1}{2})^3 = \frac{1}{8}$	1
joint	$\frac{1}{2} \times \frac{1}{8} = \frac{1}{16}$	$\frac{1}{2} \times 1 = \frac{1}{2}$
posterior probability that she's a carrier after having two unaffected boys	$\dfrac{\frac{1}{16}}{\frac{1}{16} + \frac{1}{2}} = \frac{1}{9} \approx 11\%$	

Figure 3-22   Table method of Bayes' theorem applied to example in Figure 3-19.

to phrase the question for the conditional probability is, "Now that she's had three boys, how likely is it that all would be unaffected?" For example, suppose that she had three girls. Since girls are not usually affected with hemophilia A, that would tell us nothing about her genotype. Similarly, if she had two unaffected boys and a girl, the conditional probability would be $\frac{1}{2} \times \frac{1}{2} = \frac{1}{4}$.) The rest is easy. For the joint probabilities in the third row of each column, we just multiply the previous two rows. So, for the first column, it is $\frac{1}{2} \times \frac{1}{8} = 1/16$, and for the second column it is $\frac{1}{2} \times 1 = \frac{1}{2}$. Last, we calculate the posterior probability. Remember, the denominator in this fraction is just the sum of all the possible outcomes, and this is just $\frac{1}{2} + \frac{1}{16}$. The numerator is the joint probability of the situation we are interested in (here, that she is a carrier), and is just $\frac{1}{16}$. We solve the problem with arithmetic and note that the probability that she is a carrier is 1 in 9 (about 11%). Therefore, before she had any children, the best figure we could give for her risk of being a carrier was 1 in 2. But given that it would be somewhat unlikely for a carrier to have three unaffected boys, we now calculate that her chance of being a carrier is reduced to 1 in 9. Thus, if she were to become pregnant, the likelihood that her fourth child would be a boy with hemophilia would be 1 in 9 (the probability that she is a carrier) multiplied times $\frac{1}{2}$ (the probability that she would segregate the mutant factor VIII allele to the egg during oogenesis), times $\frac{1}{2}$ (the probability of the egg being fertilized by a sperm containing a Y chromosome) = 1/36. To try to get an intuitive grasp for this question, think of the extreme case. What if she were initially at $\frac{1}{2}$ risk to be a carrier, but she had 25 unaffected boys? Of course, at this point we would begin to doubt that she inherited the mutant factor VIII allele. But, what would happen if a fourth pregnancy (or in our absurd case, a twenty-sixth pregnancy) resulted in a boy who turned out to have hemophilia A? However unlikely it may have been that she would still be a carrier and have so many unaffected boys, the birth of an affected male indicates that she is, indeed, a carrier. We would then know that her risk of having an affected boy for each future pregnancy would now be 1 (probability that she is a carrier) $\times \frac{1}{2}$ (probability of segregating the mutant factor VIII allele in the egg) $\times \frac{1}{2}$ (probability of the egg being fertilized by a sperm containing a Y chromosome) $= \frac{1}{4}$.

For those of you who prefer the branching diagram method (Fig. 3-23), we start out by knowing that there is a 1 in 2 probability that she is either a carrier or a noncarrier. If she were a noncarrier, there would be a probability of one that, if she had three boys, they would all be unaffected. If she were a carrier, every time she has a boy, there is a $\frac{1}{2}$ chance that the boy is affected or unaffected. We can cross out all the branches that lead to an affected boy, because we did not observe this to happen. When we are done drawing out the diagram, we multiply through the probabilities just as before (getting the joint probability of the table method). We then set up the fraction to give the posterior probability, just as with the table method.

Lyonization

> **Lyonization:** A term used for the random inactivation of one X chromosome in each cell of a female. It is named after Mary Lyon, who discovered X inactivation. The word usually connotes a "skewed" or "unfavorable" pattern of X chromosome inactivation, such that the female is at least partly affected for an X-linked recessive disorder.

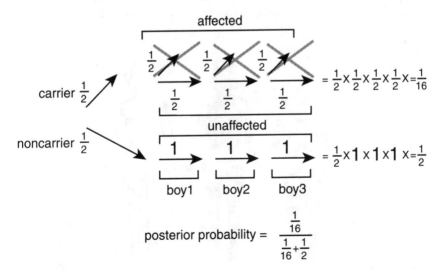

Figure 3-23 Branching diagram method of Bayes' theorem applied to example in Figure 3-19.

Females have two copies of X chromosome genes, since they have two X chromosomes. In contrast, males have only one copy of genes residing on the X chromosome, since they only have one X chromosome, and the Y chromosome, for the most part, does not have any of the same genes. The evolutionary rationale for inactivating one of the X chromosomes in females is presumably a mechanism of "dosage compensation" to ensure that both sexes have the same number of functional alleles for genes on the X chromosome. The particular X chromosome that is shut down in any particular cell will be condensed, making it visible even during the "interphase" of the mitotic cell cycle, when chromosomes are ordinarily elongated and not microscopically visible. The name for the condensed microscopic appearance of the X chromosome is the Barr body. Females ordinarily have one Barr body per cell, whereas males have zero. There are a few genes in females, however, that do escape X inactivation, even though the rest of the chromosome is shutdown. Since X chromosome inactivation is randomly distributed throughout tissues, skewing of inactivation might result in a segmental pattern of distribution of expression of the mutant gene or phenotype. As shown in Figure 3-24, some women could have some locally uneven patterns of X inactivation, merely due to random statistical variation.

Consider factor VIII in hemophilia A. Most of the factor VIII production occurs in the liver, where it is secreted into the blood stream. Extreme skewing in X inactivation is pretty uncommon for hemophilia A. This is because it does not really matter whether there is a locally uneven pattern of X inactivation in the liver cells. On balance, close to half of the hepatocytes will be producing factor VIII, and it will all get averaged out when it is secreted into the blood. A completely different situation pertains to a protein that is not secreted, but rather whose effect is local to the cell that produces it. A good example is Duchenne's

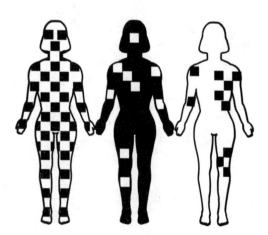

Figure 3-24   Uneven lyonization = skewed X inactivation.

muscular dystrophy. In the case of Duchenne's muscular dystrophy, the defect is in a protein, dystrophin, which is a component of the muscle contractile apparatus. If there were a skewed pattern of X inactivation in a particular muscle, then we might expect that muscle to be weak and there to be a focal pattern of weakness.

UNUSUAL FORMS OF INHERITANCE

The three standard forms of mendelian segregation still account for the majority of inherited diseases. In recent years, however, so many familial disease patterns with untraditional mendelian inheritance have been discovered that they can no longer be ignored in an introductory discussion. Although most remain rare, these diseases attract a lot of interest because they tend to be the exceptions that "prove the rule" of mendelian inheritance.

Mitochondrial

Maternally inherited transmission occurs when the defective gene is encoded in the mitochondrial genome (Fig. 3-25). The mitochondria are subcellular organelles in which aerobic energy metabolism occurs. They are inherited exclusively from the cytoplasm of the oocyte during the formation of the zygote and are, therefore, exclusively maternal in origin. Mitochondria contain their own circular, (approximately) sixteen-thousand basepair genome, DNA and RNA polymerases, and protein translation apparatus including ribosomes and tRNA. The genetic code is also slightly different between mitochondrial and nuclear genomes. Many mitochondrial proteins are encoded by the mitochondrial DNA; some mitochondrial proteins, however, are encoded by the nuclear genome and are inherited in a mendelian fashion. Most children of an affected female are usually affected, to varying degrees, whereas children of an affected male are never

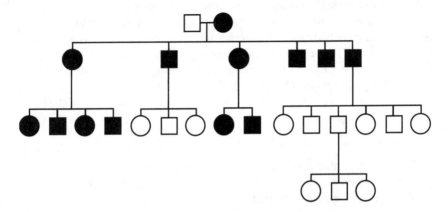

Figure 3-25   Example: Mitochondrial inheritance.

affected. Examples of mitochondrially inherited diseases include myoclonus epilepsy with ragged red fibers (MERRF), mitochondrial myopathy/encephalopathy/lactic-acidosis/stroke-like episodes (MELAS), and Kearns-Sayre syndrome. These diseases tend to have some degree of clinical overlap, and the first two are pretty much as described by their lengthy names. MERRF and MELAS result from a variety of different mutations in mitochondrially encoded tRNA molecules. Kearns-Sayre syndrome is characterized by weakness of the muscles of the orbit coordinating eye movement and results from large-scale mitochondrial deletions. Recently, some inherited forms of common diseases have been found to result from maternally inherited mitochondrial mutations, including some instances of diabetes mellitus, cardiomyopathies, and predisposition to deafness on exposure to toxic concentrations of aminoglycoside antibiotics. "Somatic" mutations (non-inherited and acquired after fertilization, birth, or with aging) in mitochondrial DNA have been associated with aging, and have been proposed as one mechanism contributing to aging.

In mitochondrial inheritance, the disease can only be inherited from the mother, and usually all of an affected mother's children are affected. However, sometimes children can escape inheriting a mitochondrial disorder or can be affected to variable degrees, depending upon how the mutation is distributed within the population of hundreds of mitochondria inherited from the mother—a concept known as "heteroplasmy."

Imprinting

With imprinting, inheritance of a trait occurs only from one parent. This is because the particular gene is only expressed from either the maternally or paternally inherited allele. The most extreme examples are hydatiform mole and ovarian teratoma, each considered a malignancy. The former usually results from fertilization of a polar body by an X chromosome containing sperm; it is all placenta without embryo. The latter results from an egg spontaneously becoming diploid and acting as if it has been fertilized; it gives rise to embryonic differentiation, but no placenta. Both are 46, XX and, therefore, chromosomally identical. The only difference between these two (and a normal female conceptus) are the handful of imprinted genes.

For rare, imprinted genes, gene expression occurs from only one parent's allele. The chosen parental allele is constant from one person to the next for all of the few, known imprinted genes.

Prader-Willi and Angelman syndrome are well-known examples of diseases that result from oppositely imprinted genes in the same region of chromosome 15.

In the Prader-Willi and Angelman syndromes, an identical "microdeletion" of a critical region of chromosome 15 will have a different phenotype depending on from which parent it is inherited. Prader-Willi syndrome evidently can only result from a deletion incorporating a cluster of contiguous genes. It is a "contiguous gene deletion syndrome" (we will discuss this in further detail later). Prader-Willi syndrome is characterized in the neonatal period clinically by failure to thrive, hypotonia, and mild to moderate mental retardation. Later on in childhood, these individuals have difficulty with satiety and have an enormous appetite for food. Consequently, individuals with Prader-Willi syndrome become quite obese. The oppositely imprinted homolog of Prader-Willi syndrome is Angelman syndrome and consists of a somewhat small body habitus with severe mental retardation and a marionette-like scissoring gait (unfortunately described as the "happy puppet" syndrome). Prader-Willi results from paternal inheritance of the deleted segment, while Angelman syndrome results from maternal inheritance. While the apparently identical deletion can produce either Prader-Willi or Angelman syndrome, depending on from which parent it was inherited, the Angelman syndrome can also result from just a single point mutation in a single gene. The hypothetical pedigree given in Figure 3-26 illustrates identical family structures, but structures in which the gene segregates with an opposite imprinting pattern in the two families.

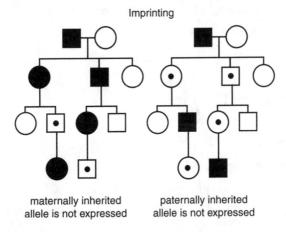

Figure 3-26   **Hypothetical example contrasting opposite imprinting patterns.**

The significance of imprinting remains unclear. It has been noted, however, that most of the handful of genes that are known to be imprinted are generally responsible for growth and have effects also in fetal life. Some have argued that this represents a molecular battle of the sexes, in which the father imprints these genes in an "on" position. This is to be sure that they are expressed in the conception that he has fathered so that he will have big, healthy kids. The mother imprints these genes in the "off" position, so that her fetus will not grow too large and endanger her own well-being. From the cold-hearted evolutionary perspective of males who often mate with multiple females, the payoff of big children might be worth the gamble of occasionally killing off the child's mother.

Germline mosaicism

Germline mosaicism occurs when the original mutation arises post-zygotically in the affected parent such that only a fraction of his or her cells contain the mutation. In particular, the germ line cells giving rise to the gametes do contain the mutation, but the mutation is in such minority in the rest of the tissues of the body that is does not produce a recognizable phenotype (Fig. 3-27). It explains the recurrence of autosomal dominant disease in a family with two unaffected parents. It is best documented in osteogenesis imperfecta, an autosomal dominant disorder of collagen producing brittle bones prone to recurrent breakage. One particularly striking case of germline mosaicism was found when a man without osteogenesis imperfecta fathered two children with the disease by two different women. The collagen mutation could be molecularly identified and was identical in both the children, but appeared absent from DNA extracted from peripheral white blood cells in the father. However, individual hairs were plucked from his head and then PCR amplified and subjected to mutational analysis. As it turned out, some of the hair shafts had the mutation and others did not—demonstrating mosaicism down to the level of individual cells on the scalp.

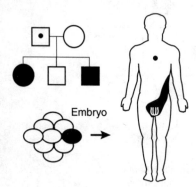

Figure 3-27   Germline mosaicism.

Some recent evidence indicates that germline mosaicism might be a surprisingly common phenomenon, although, for the purposes of genetic counseling, we generally ignore it, except in those rare situations in which we have explicit evidence to the contrary.

Germline mosaicism should be considered as a possible explanation for a couple in which neither parent is affected, yet have more than one child with a highly penetrant autosomal dominant illness.

Autosomal dominant nonviable

There are mutations in some genes in which the phenotypic effects are so severe that they would result in a non-viable pregnancy. Consequently, these are only seen in a mosaic state in affected individuals, in which the mutation is confined to a small patch of tissue (Fig. 3-28). The mutations are somatic, arising post-zygotically in one cell in the embryo. The most well-characterized example is McCune-Albright syndrome. McCune-Albright syndrome is virtually never inherited, as would be expected with such a disease, and results from activating mutations in the alpha subunit of the stimulatory G protein that regulates intracellular signaling. Clinically, McCune-Albright is characterized by multiple endocrine tumors that represent somatic foci of constitutively activated cells. These initially over-express a particular hormone and then, sometimes, progress to a malignant state.

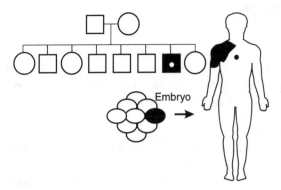

Figure 3-28   Autosomal dominant nonviable.

MUTATION

•

- **New Mutation**
- **Fitness**
- **Haldane's Rule**
- **The Origins of Mutation**

  Allelic Heterogeneity

  Allelic Disorders

  Locus Heterogeneity

  Phenocopy

  Heterozygote Advantage

•   •   •   •   •   •   •   •   •   •   •   •   •

NEW MUTATION

What are the explanations for the pedigree shown in Fig. 4-1, in which two unaffected parents give birth to a child with achondroplasia? Achondroplasia is an autosomal dominant disease of short-limbed dwarfism resulting from a single basepair mutation leading to amino acid substitution in the fibroblast growth factor receptor 3 (FGFR3) gene. In this family, we have two normal stature and unaffected parents who have a child with achondroplasia. We can exclude incomplete penetrance in the parents, because achondroplasia is completely penetrant. We should consider three possible explanations. First, non-paternity is always a possibility. No one knows the true incidence of non-paternity, but it is probably on the order of 1% to 5%. In this particular example, the unknown father would

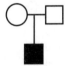

Figure 4-1   Example: Anchondroplasia.

also have to have achondroplasia, however. A second possible explanation, which we have already discussed, is germline mosaicism. Germline mosaicism has been documented to occur for achondroplasia, but it is a rare phenomenon. At this point, we have no reason to invoke it as a consideration in this family, but if this couple had two children with achondroplasia, this would be the most probable explanation. The third possibility, however, given the current pedigree with just one affected child, is the most probable, and that is, that the child represents a new mutation (also known as "de novo" mutation). In other words, the mutation occurred for the first time in this family's history in the affected child.

Whenever a child with a highly penetrant autosomal dominant disease is born to two unaffected parents, the possibility of new mutation or nonpaternity should be considered (in that order). When a second unaffected child is born to the same couple, germline mosaicism also becomes a possibility.

Typically, the mutation would occur in a gamete (egg or sperm) that gave rise to the individual. The mutation could also occur in the zygote or very early post-zygotically such that it was present in the majority of the cells of the embryo. If it occurred many cell divisions later than that in the embryo, it would be distributed in a mosaic fashion. New mutations represent about a third of all cases of achondroplasia, and, therefore, a family like this is not uncommon. It turns out that for achondroplasia, all of the new mutations occur on the paternal chromosome and appear to be associated with advanced paternal age.

In general, advanced paternal age is associated with an increased risk for new mutations in a single gene, mendelian disorder. As we will discuss later, advanced maternal age is associated with a risk for chromosomal disorders resulting from meiotic non-disjunction.

FITNESS

For serious autosomal dominant illness, new mutations account for 100%. Why should it be so high? The answer is because the "fitness" (relative success at having offspring) is reduced. Individuals affected with serious disease either die before reproductive age, are sterile, or are not successful in attracting a mate. Thus, in order to account for the constant disease incidence in the population over time, the alleles lost to lethal events must be replaced by new mutations.

For example, heterozygous mutations in the protease neutrophil elastase are the most common cause of congenital neutropenia. Neutropenic individuals have a near absence of circulating neutrophils (phagocytic white blood cells) and usually succumb to opportunistic infections or are otherwise too sick to become parents. Consequently, nearly all elastase mutations newly arise, and there is seldom a family history of neutropenia.

HALDANE'S RULE

A simplified extrapolation of Haldane's rule basically says that one third of all persons affected with a severe X-linked recessive disease will represent new mutations, without a prior family history.

Let us look at the situation in diseases that are lethal, where fitness is zero. All the alleles in an affected male are lost in just one generation and must be replaced with new mutations to ensure a constant incidence of the disease over time. Since one third of all X chromosomes in the population are in males, one third of all lethal alleles should be new mutations. In fact, this is observed to be true for Duchenne's muscular dystrophy and some other illnesses. (Haldane also had another rule about inter-species hybrids being sterile, but we are not concerned with that here.)

THE ORIGINS OF MUTATION

Mutation: A change in DNA sequence, usually conferring a deleterious effect.
Polymorphism: DNA sequence difference, usually of no pathologic significance.

A variety of different mutations are possible. A "point mutation" generally refers to a single base substitution, insertion, or deletion. Sometimes, a point mutation has no deleterious effect. This is the usual case if it occurs in an intron (away from the splice donor or acceptor sites) or outside of the coding sequence. Base substitutions that do not change the amino acid specified by the triplet codon are also inconsequential. In these cases, this is not really a mutation, per se, but rather a "polymorphism" of no particular significance. Polymorphisms can be used to differentiate the DNA sequences of two particular alleles but are otherwise inconsequential. On the other hand, a single base insertion or deletion in the coding region of a gene almost always has a deleterious effect since it results in a "frame shift," which alters the reading frame and changes almost every following amino acid. Frame shifts often lead to the reading of an inappropriate out-of-frame termination codon and lead to the appearance of a prematurely truncated protein. Single base substitutions in the coding region that alter an amino acid can either represent a mutation, and alter the function of the protein, or they can be of no consequence.

Often during the course of genetic testing, a new single base substitution resulting in an alteration of the amino acid sequence of the protein may be discovered, but it is difficult to determine whether this represents a mutation or polymorphism. Larger scale mutations, like lengthy deletions, insertions, or inversions of a sequence, are more likely to have deleterious effects, but since only a minority of the genome actually contains genes, even these are often of no particular significance

ALLELIC HETEROGENEITY

> **Allelic heterogeneity:** Occurs when multiple types of mutations in a given gene can account for the inheritance of the same disorder in different families.

One example is cystic fibrosis, where about 70% of the mutant alleles in the population are the ΔF508. The remaining 30% represent a collection of different mutations. The different mutations can account for interfamilial differences in expressivity for a genetic disorder.

In contrast, in some circumstances, all individuals with a particular disease have exactly the same mutation (or at most, just a few different mutations). This occurs when there are "founder effects," such as when all individuals affected with the disorder are descended from a common affected ancestor. This is seen in diseases common among a particular ethnic group, such as Tay-Sachs disease in Ashkenazi (eastern European) Jews. Tay-Sachs is an autosomal recessive, early childhood onset, neurodegenerative disease caused by loss of function in the neuraminidase gene. Neuraminidase functions in the lysosome to break down sphingolipids. When not functioning, the lysosomes become packed with cellular debris, and there is neuronal toxicity. The disease is inexorable and leads to death usually well before puberty. During the Middle Ages, the European Jewish population was decimated, and it has been estimated that as few as several thousand individuals contributed to the modern day Diaspora. Consequently, any recessive mutation present in a carrier state in one of those limited number of ancestors may be represented in a large number of their descendants today. The same phenomenon is true for other relatively isolated ethnic groups. Inherited diseases with characteristically limited ethnic distributions can be found among French Canadians, various Scandinavian populations, particular Arab populations, the Eskimo, and other racial groups. (On the other hand, Tay-Sachs is an interesting example where there has been selection for the heterozygote carrier state, presumably as a consequence of some unknown selective advantage, that we will discuss shortly.)

ALLELIC DISORDERS

> **Allelic disorders:** This is an extreme example of how different mutations in the same gene can cause divergent phenotypes, in which there are actually two different diseases caused by the same gene.

One example of a pair of allelic disorders is multiple endocrine neoplasia 2 and Hirschsprung's megacolon, both of which result from mutation in the RET gene. You will hear more about multiple endocrine neoplasia 2 (in the chapter on cancer genetics), an autosomal dominant family cancer syndrome characterized by predisposition to medullary thyroid carcinoma, pheochromocytoma, and parathyroid adenoma. It is definitely quite distinct from Hirschsprung's megacolon, an etiologically heterogeneous disorder resulting from a failure of formation of the enteric neurons of the colon with loss of intestinal motility.

LOCUS HETEROGENEITY

> **Locus heterogeneity:** the same disease can be caused by mutations in different genes. For example, there are multiple genes that can cause either polycystic kidney disease, tuberous sclerosis, or spinal cerebellar ataxia.

> **To summarize:** In allelic heterogeneity, there are multiple alleles, all producing more or less the same disease, for a particular gene. In genetic heterogeneity, more than one gene can cause the same disease. Allelic disorders result when different mutations in the same gene cause different diseases.

PHENOCOPY

> **Phenocopy:** This represents the occurrence of a genetic disease that, in any particular individual, may not be due to genetic causes.

For example, porphyria cutanea tarda, a metabolic defect in heme synthesis, leading to hepatic insufficiency and rash, can be inherited or can be acquired from exposure to drugs, alcohol, and other undefined factors. Thus, even if an individual is a member of a family in which other people have inherited porphyria, it is still possible that he or she can get the disease as a result of other causes, even without inheriting the gene. Phenocopies are a particular problem when sorting out mendelian inheritance of disorders that usually occur in a common, sporadic, non-inherited form, such as breast cancer.

HETEROZYGOTE ADVANTAGE

Selective pressures operate differently for autosomal recessive diseases than they do for dominant diseases. A low fitness for a recessive disease has little effect on removing a disease allele from the population, as it would for a dominant disease. This is because most of the alleles are hidden in unaffected heterozygotes. On the other hand, selective pressures can influence the heterozygote population. If the heterozygotes have a selective advantage compared to those who are homozygous for normal alleles, the frequency of the disease allele will increase. Since heterozygotes are far more common than homozygotes, for any given disease allele, the benefit to the frequent heterozygote population may be more than enough to make up for any deleterious effect in the infrequent homozygous population. This is the reason why sickle cell disease and thalassemia are so common in the regions of the world with malaria. Sickle cell anemia is an autosomal recessive disease resulting from the substitution of valine for glutamic acid at the 6th position of the beta chain of hemoglobin. Heterozygous carriers of the sickle cell trait are relatively resistant to malarial infection and complications, with the downside being sickle cell anemia in the less common homozygotes. The same is thought to be true of the maintenance of recessive alleles for cystic fibrosis. There is good evidence that individuals heterozygous for cystic fibrosis mutations are relatively resistant to cholera and salmonella enteritis.

The heterozygote advantage results from the fact that $2pq \gg q^2$, from the Hardy-Weinberg law, and explains the high carrier frequency for certain autosomal recessive disease alleles that confer disease resistance in a heterozygote state.

Tay-Sachs disease demonstrates both founder effects and heterozygote selection in the Ashkenazi Jewish population. We know this because there are two common mutations present in the Ashkenazi population at a relatively high carrier frequency. If it were just a seemingly random founder effect, we should not expect there to be two different alleles, so we infer that there was a specific selective advantage. Many theories have been advanced, including heterozygote selection for resistance to tuberculosis (a presumably common disease of those crowded into the close confines of the ghetto), but these remain unproven.

Carrier selection also occurs for sex-linked recessive disease, as in the case of glucose-6-phosphate dehydrogenase (G6PD) deficiency, which follows a geo-ethnic distribution similar to that of sickle cell disease and appears to confer similar resistance to malarial infection and its complications. G6PD participates in the hexose monophosphate shunt of glycolysis. A deficiency of G6PD activity results in hemolytic anemia upon exposure to oxidants, including sulfa antibiotics, antimalarials, and fava beans. In fact, since both Lyonization and carrier selection apply in the case of G6PD deficiency, one can make a striking observation in the peripheral blood smear of female carriers infected with malaria. If the smear is stained to histochemically detect G6PD, then Lyonization will be detectable at the level of a single cell—some erythrocytes will express G6PD and others will not. Interestingly enough, the malarial parasites will be seen preferentially in the red cells that express G6PD and will be relatively scarce in the red cells that lack G6PD activity. Ironically, G6PD first became widely recognized when African-American GI's serving in Korea in the 1950s fell ill after receiving prophylactic malarial therapy.

GENETIC TESTING

•

• • • • • • • • • • • •

DIRECT TESTING

For many genetic diseases, the responsible gene has been identified, and it is possible to molecularly examine the gene for mutations. Direct testing refers to direct identification of the DNA sequence change by DNA sequencing, or other methods, such as Southern blot (best for detecting deletions) or PCR assay. The main advantage of direct testing is that only the patient needs to be studied. (You do not necessarily need to get DNA from other family members, some of whom may be non-cooperative or dead.) On the other hand, even when the gene responsible for the disease is uniquely known, it is sometimes difficult to find the exact mutation, and having knowledge of the mutation in a previously studied relative, can expedite testing substantially.

Direct testing refers to direct mutational analysis of a gene causing a particular disease. When this is not possible, because the gene has not been identified, or the gene is too large and there is too much allelic heterogeneity, then indirect testing in the form of linkage analysis is performed.

INDIRECT TESTING AND THE CONCEPT OF LINKAGE ANALYSIS

Indirect testing is used either when the gene is not known but linkage with a genetic marker has been established, or when the gene is known but the mutation cannot be found. Linkage analysis is also the primary strategy through which most human disease genes have been discovered.

Linkage is a difficult concept to understand, so we will go through it in a step-wise approach. Let us consider the simplest case of linkage. Suppose that a gene for a particular disease is deleted, and the deletion is so large that this chromosomal aberration is visible microscopically through a karyotype (more on this later in the cytogenetics chapter). In this case, we can follow the inheritance of that gene quite easily; whoever has the chromosomal abnormality must have the mutation. The aberrant marker chromosome and the disease will both segregate together in a mendelian pattern throughout the family. In fact, this hardly ever happens.

So, let us take the next-simplest case. Now, we have a disease gene that resides on a chromosome with some other microscopically visible abnormality that has nothing to do with the disease. (Yes, there are benign structural chromosome variants distinguishable by staining and other means that do not result in disease, although they, too, are uncommon.) Remember, the disease gene is located some distance from this marker region on the chromosome, and the mutation does not have anything to do with the alteration that gives rise to the marker characteristic of the chromosome. Most of the time, the marker region of this chromosome and the disease will always segregate together, and we can predict that whoever inherits this variant chromosome will also inherit the disease gene. But why is this not true all of the time? Because as long as the marker is some distance from the actual disease gene, there is an opportunity for a recombination event during meiosis in the formation of a gamete. When that recombination occurs, the actual disease gene will move onto the normal parental chromosome homolog, and the marker region and the disease will no longer segregate with each other. The probability that the marker and the disease will segregate during meiosis is solely a function of the distance between the two on the chromosome

(Fig. 5-1). If the marker and the disease gene are close by, they will hardly ever segregate from one another. Recall that there is approximately one recombination event per chromosome arm per meiosis. So, if the marker and the disease gene are on opposite ends of a chromosome, there will almost always be a recombination event between them and they will never demonstrate linkage. That is, they will segregate together with only a 1 in 2 probability at each meiosis.

> The greater the distance between any two loci on a chromosome, whether they be two genes, or a gene and a marker, the greater the probability of a meiotic recombination. In other words, recombination frequency is generally proportional to the physical distance between the two loci.

> The tightness of linkage is defined by recombination frequency: 1 centi-Morgan (cM) = 1% probability of recombination per meiosis. In general, 1 cM ≈ one million basepairs (megabase) of DNA.

It is very rare to find a chromosomal aberration that can be detected microscopically and be used as a marker to follow disease inheritance. Consequently, researchers began to look for molecular markers. In early studies in the 1950s and 1960s, markers were not even DNA based—they were biochemical markers based on blood groups and HLA. The assumption was that these serum and cellular proteins had to be encoded by a particular gene on a particular chromosome. If that gene was located nearby on the same chromosome as the disease gene, it was expected that the marker and the disease would co-segregate within a family. Since the number of such biochemical markers was limited, only a few chromosomes could be scrutinized for linkage; and the chromosome location of these markers was not even known. Amazingly, these researchers operated on the faith that the theory of genes was correct and that someday this would all be worked out at some tractable molecular level. Subsequently it has been shown that HLA resides on chromosome 6, the ABO blood group on chromosome 9, the rh blood group on chromosome 1, and so forth.

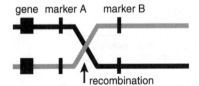

gene marker A   marker B

recombination

Figure 5-1
If gene and marker are nearby (A), recombination is less likely to occur between them. If gene and marker are far apart (B), recombination is more likely to occur between them.

RFLPs

To improve the utility of linkage studies, researchers beginning in the 1980s proposed the use of anonymous DNA markers. In the early days of DNA-based linkage, RFLPs (restriction fragment length polymorphisms) emerged (Fig. 5-2). RFLPs are based on the premise that for some marker sequences adjacent to the gene of interest, there will be inter-individual differences in the length of the sequence between two restriction cleavage sites (resulting from single base changes that abolish an intervening restriction site). The technique was somewhat cumbersome, because Southern blots were required for detection, and the markers were not very "informative." For most RFLPs, there were just two or three different alleles recognizable in the population for any given marker. The more alleles for a given marker in the population, the more likely an individual will be heterozygous and genotypically distinct from his or her mate, thus allowing for the outcomes of the mating to be uniquely genotyped. Markers with a greater number of alleles present in the population are usually more informative.

MICROSATELLITE MARKERS

Today, almost all linkage studies are performed with PCR-based "microsatellite" markers derived from polymorphic repetitive sequences, usually of variable numbers of dinucleotide CA repeats or tetranucleotide repeats of other sequences (Fig.5-3). These markers represent a technical advance over RFLPs because they use PCR (hence rapidity and small quantities of DNA) and because they are highly informative, typically with multiple alleles within the population. Since a good marker may have a dozen or more alleles in the population, it is somewhat unlikely that a parent will be homozygous for two alleles or that both parents will have a common allele between them. This helps to differentiate the outcomes of matings quite readily and allows for more informative testing.

It is important to remember that in most families, there will be different alleles of the marker locus segregating with the disease gene. It is easy to see why this is true. For families whose mutations demonstrate allelic heterogeneity, the

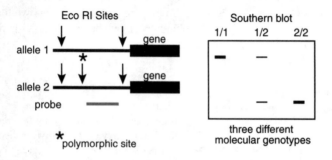

Figure 5-2 RFLPs.

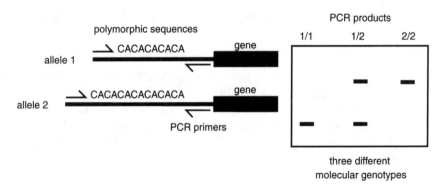

Figure 5-3   Microsatellite markers.

mutations must have arisen at different points in time on different and unrelated ancestral chromosomes. Nevertheless, this is still usually true, even with families sharing a common ancestral mutation coming from a relatively isolated ethnic group. This is because, over time, there are enough meioses to shuffle around almost all areas of the chromosome. Only the most tightly linked loci on a chromosome will not have had a recombination event occur between them over the generations. Thus, in each family, a unique analysis must be performed to first correlate the inheritance of a particular marker allele with the disease phenotype. Only when this is established can the linkage analysis be used to make any diagnostic predictions within a family.

SNPs

In the near future, there will likely be a third generation of markers, known as "single nucleotide polymorphisms," or SNPs (pronounced "snips"). Single base-pair differences between individuals are pretty common and easy to find, in contrast to RFLPs and dinucleotide or tetranucleotide repeats, which take a bit of effort to develop and are spaced somewhat infrequently in the genome. In fact, on average, SNPs can be found about every thousand basepairs in the genome. The disadvantage to SNPs is that there can be a maximum of just four alleles in the population for any given SNP (i.e., just an A, C, T, or G at a single position). One great advantage, however, is that SNPs can be screened by high throughput hybridization methods. Leading edge research in hybridization technology employs "DNA chips," wafers with high density arrays of oligonucleotides capable of hybridizing or not hybridizing to certain SNPs. What is envisioned is that an individual's total genomic DNA can be fluorescently labeled, momentarily placed on a chip to hybridize, and the resulting pattern of spots detected nearly immediately using light signals. Considerably more markers could be rapidly screened, although the information content per each marker would be less and computationally sophisticated approaches would be required to decode the information.

Three types of DNA markers have been developed for linkage testing. RFLPs are the labor intensive, obsolete technology of the past. Microsatellite markers are presently in use and lend themselves well to large-scale automation. SNPs are an emerging technology that promises to revolutionize the genetic analysis of large numbers of people, thereby providing the power to study the effects of weaker genes in complex traits.

LOD SCORE ANALYSIS

A methodical process of establishing linkage ever more tightly and searching for mutations in all the genes found in the delimited region defines the "positional cloning" strategy, which has been used to clone most of the identified disease-causing human genes. The competing approach is the "candidate gene" method, in which biologically plausible candidate genes are evaluated as the cause of an inherited disease without first performing any kind of linkage study. This approach usually fails. In contrast, the number of human disease genes now successfully identified through positional cloning methods has grown so large, and continues to expand on a nearly weekly basis, that it is beyond listing.

Most positional cloning projects begin with a "genome-wide screen" for linkage. Researchers preferably begin with a large collection of DNA samples taken from families inheriting a particular disease where the chromosomal location of the responsible disease gene is unknown. Several hundred DNA markers, usually microsatellite markers in most contemporary approaches, are assembled from regularly spaced genetic intervals, typically 10 to 20 cM, from each chromosome. Each marker is then scrutinized to determine if its inheritance co-segregates with the disease phenotype. The most commonly used statistical test of association between inheritance of a marker and disease phenotype is the LOD score.

LOD score: A log of the odds (LOD) in favor of linkage of a genetic marker to a phenotype as opposed to non-linkage (random segregation). A LOD score of 3 (interpreted as 1000:1 in favor of a conditional probability of linkage) is the arbitrarily accepted standard for linkage for an autosomal disease. (For reasons related to Baye's theorm, a LOD score of 3 corresponds to a p value of about 0.05 that the null hypothesis of no linkage is true, when a typical genome-wide screen for linkage is undertaken.)

Let us actually calculate a LOD score. In the following example of an auto-somal dominant disease, we assume the marker to be so tightly linked to the dis-ease locus that we can ignore the possibility of recombination. Note that this hypothetical marker in the pedigree illustrated in Figure 5-4 is "fully informative" for all crosses (i.e. every husband and wife pair has four different alleles for this marker between them, although markers can be fully informative with fewer than four alleles in the mating pair) and all the family members are available. We have two affected first cousins and they have the same allele (number 1) for the marker, as does each cousin's affected parent and their common affected grand-father. To calculate the LOD score, we need to figure out how likely it is that they would both inherit this marker by chance (the denominator). The probability of transmission of the marker at each generation is 1 in 2. Thus, by multiplying inde-pendent probabilities, there is a 1 in 4 chance of one cousin inheriting allele num-ber 1 from the affected grandfather and a 1 in 4 chance of the other cousin inheriting the allele from the affected grandfather. So, there is a 1 in 16 chance of both cousins inheriting allele number 1. Now, the numerator is the probability of inheriting allele number 1 if it is linked to disease; this is easy and is just 1. So, the LOD score is the $\log\left(1/\frac{1}{16}\right) = \log 16 = 1.20$. Note that it takes a family of at least 10 individuals to map a gene with significance by the LOD score method, since $\log\left(1/(\frac{1}{2})^{10}\right) \approx 3.0$. In reality, however, most studies are conducted with far larger numbers of individuals and are facilitated by the fact that LOD scores from one family can be added to the LOD scores of another family when performing a research study to hunt for a gene.

This seems pretty easy, but the following situations almost always occur and complicate linkage analysis.

1. Some people in the family are dead or refuse to participate. Genotypes must therefore, be inferred, and cannot always be done so uniquely with the infor-mation that is provided.
2. Markers are not always informative to differentiate the outcome of every mating. If one affected person is homozygous for a particular allele, it is not possible to determine if that marker segregates with the phenotype.

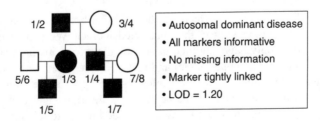

Figure 5-4   Calculation of a LOD score.

3. The marker is some distance from the actual gene, and there is, thus, the possibility of recombination at every mating.
4. Many diseases are incompletely penetrant or display age-dependent penetrance. Therefore, it is not always so easy to specify whether someone who has inherited the gene is fortuitously unaffected or just has not lived long enough to develop symptoms of the disease.
5. Some individuals may represent phenocopies, who develop the disease that the rest of the family inherits sporadically, rather than on a hereditary basis.
6. In some families, the disease, especially when common, can be introduced a second time from someone who marries into the family.
7. Finally, when studying more than one family, genetic heterogeneity is possible, so that some families will link to one locus and others families to other loci, thus giving potentially conflicting results.

So, linkage testing is used for research purposes to find genes in the first place and in a few individual clinical situations when direct mutational analysis cannot be used. Disadvantages are that such studies require the cooperation of relatives, are more involved, and frequently do not give a black or white answer. Let us look at some particular examples of linkage testing and see how these pitfalls crop up.

The following pedigrees illustrate a highly penetrant autosomal dominant disease. We assume that a prior research linkage study in large families with the disease has determined the chromosomal location of the gene to a high probability (LOD score > 3). Now, we wish to apply that research result to a particular clinical situation in which we attempt prenatal diagnosis. Remember that most modern markers have multiple alleles within the population, but we limit ourselves here to a marker with two alleles to simplify things. The two different alleles are represented by two different sized PCR bands amplifying polymorphic microsatellite markers tightly linked to the disease gene. We call one allele the "lower" allele, and the other, the "upper" allele. Assume that the fetus's DNA has been sampled by amniocentesis or chorionic villus sampling. (Both methods will be discussed in greater detail later.) The pedigrees are drawn to align each individual with a corresponding lane on the gel.

What is the risk for the pregnancy in each of these two families illustrated in Figure 5-5? In the pedigree on the left, it is 100%. We see here that the son inherited the disease from his affected father and that both have in common the upper allele, which is lacking in the unaffected mother. We conclude that the affected son could only have inherited the upper allele from his father (since his mother does not have an upper allele) and that the lower allele must have come from the unaffected mother. The fetus inherited the upper allele—linked to the disease—and will be affected. In the pedigree on the right, the fetus has a 0% probability of inheriting the disease. Again, we see linkage to the upper allele in both the affected father and son, but the fetus inherited a lower allele from each

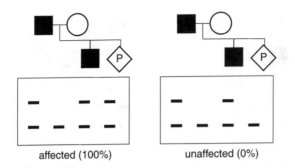

affected (100%)   unaffected (0%)

Figure 5-5   What is the risk for this pregnancy?
Assume autosomal dominant disease with two alleles in the population, distinguishable by a tightly linked marker.

parent. (The fetus did not get the upper allele from the father, so the fetus had to get the lower allele and is homozygous for the lower allele.)

What is the risk for the pregnancy illustrated in Figure 5-6? This is uninformative and we cannot refine the risk any further by testing, other than stating that, since it is autosomal dominant, it will still be 50%. Each parent is homozygous for the lower allele and the two offspring must be necessarily homozygous for these two alleles.

What is the risk for the pregnancy shown in Figure 5-7? In this case, we can differentiate the unaffected mother's allele, and we can see that both the affected son and the fetus inherited the lower allele from the mother. Unfortunately, this does not help us. The affected father is homozygous for the lower allele, so it is still not possible to determine linkage, and again, the testing is uninformative.

What is the risk for the pregnancy shown in Figure 5-8? This is a case where both parents are heterozygous for the two alleles. The fetus inherits a lower allele from each parent and is homozygous for the lower allele. However, it is not possible to tell whether the disease segregates with the upper or lower allele, because the "phase" is undetermined for the affected son. The son could have inherited the upper allele from his father and the lower allele from his mother; or, he could

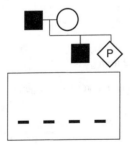

Figure 5-6   What is the risk for this pregnancy?

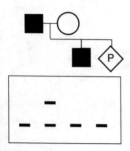

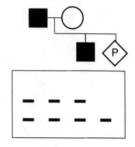

Figure 5-7 What is the risk for this pregnancy?

Figure 5-8 What is the risk for this pregnancy?

have inherited the lower allele from his father and the upper allele from his mother. Because we cannot distinguish which happened, we cannot determine which allele is linked to the gene, and, once again, the testing is uninformative.

Now let us look at another example, just like the first one, except that now we say that the marker is 10 cM distant from the gene (Fig. 5-9). This means that there is a 10% probability of recombination between the marker and the gene with each meiosis. Again, it looks like the disease segregates with the upper allele between affected father and son in the paternal meiosis that gave rise to the son. However, in the paternal meiosis leading to the sperm that produced the fetus, there was a 10% chance that the mutant allele for the disease gene recombined onto the opposite, lower allele. So, even though the fetus inherited the upper allele from the father, there is a 10% chance that there was a recombination placing the mutant disease allele on a paternal chromosome with the lower marker. The result is that there is only a 90% probability that the fetus is affected.

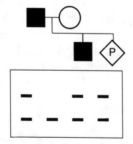

same as first case, except marker is 10 CM distant from gene

probability affected = 100% - probability of recombination between marker and the gene

= 100% - 10% = 90%

Figure 5-9 Effect of recombination.

The last example is similar (Fig. 5-10), except that we introduce genetic heterogeneity. Ninety percent of families result from mutation on the chromosome we are looking at, but 10% of families have the disease as a result of a mutation in a different gene on a different chromosome. In this care, we are confident that the fetus inherited the same paternal allele as the affected son; however, we are only 90% certain that this is the locus causing the disease in this family.

Linkage testing can fail as a consequence of insufficiently informative markers, markers that are insufficiently close enough to the locus of the disease (and, thereby, having a high rate of recombination between the marker and disease gene), and genetic heterogeneity, in which the wrong locus is tested for linkage.

HAPLOTYPE ANALYSIS

Haplotype: A group of alleles from closely linked loci that are usually inherited as a unit. Haplotype analysis can be used in genetic testing and positional cloning to determine if affected individuals inherited a common chromosomal region.

Let us examine the inheritance of the highly penetrant autosomal dominant disease illustrated in this example (Fig. 5-11). Genotypes have been determined

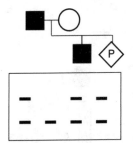

return to tightly linked marker, but for
this disease 10% of families are due to
mutations in a gene on a different chromosome

Figure 5-10   Effect of genetic heterogeneity.

for six highly polymorphic markers that, as shown, are spaced equally across the length of the chromosome. All affected individuals have inherited a common chromosomal region (spanning from marker two to marker four) from individual number one. In the second generation, it can be seen that individual number three inherited the entire "A" haplotype from individual one. (The "A" haplotype consists of alleles 16, 4, 4, 6, 2, and 7 for markers one through six, respectively.) Individual three's unaffected brother, individual seven, inherited the opposite "a" haplotype (comprised of alleles 1, 4, 5, 8, 1, and 3 for markers one through six, respectively). Individual five also inherited the "A" haplotype from individual one; however, there was a recombination (here denoted with an "x") between

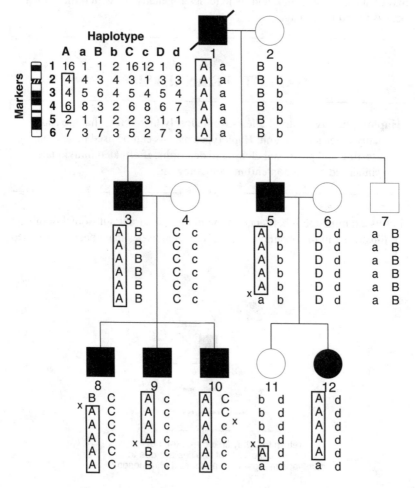

Figure 5-11 Haplotype analysis.

marker five and six in the paternal meiosis that recombined the "a" haplotype onto the chromosome containing the "A" haplotype for the distal segment of the long arm. The three affected children of individual three, persons eight, nine, and ten, also inherited portions of the "A" haplotype. Again, there is recombination in the paternal meiosis, which gave rise to individuals eight and nine, between the first and second markers and the fourth and fifth markers, respectively. There is also recombination in the maternal meiosis (individual four) for person ten, between markers five and six of the "C" and "c" haplotypes. The children of individual five show similar patterns. The unaffected daughter, person eleven, inherited most of the "b" haplotype from individual five. Again, we see that there was a recombination in the paternal meiosis between markers four and five in person eleven. The net result is that individual eleven now has one chromosome containing portions of haplotype "b" (markers one through four), haplotype "A" (marker five), and haplotype "a" (marker six). Note that this single chromosome now has regions coming from three different great-grandparents. The "A" and "a" haplotypes originated from grandparent individual one (and, in turn, each of those haplotypes came from individual one's parents, who are not shown on the pedigree). The "b" haplotype came from grandparent individual two (who, in turn, inherited this from one of her parents). Individual twelve inherited the "A/a" recombinant haplotype, without further recombination, from his father (person five) and a non-recombinant "d" haplotype from his mother (person six). Thus, it can be seen that if we are supposing that the gene responsible for the illness in this family resides on this chromosome, it must localize between markers two and four, since all affected individuals have inherited this region in common, but none of the unaffected individuals at risk for inheriting the disease inherited this portion of the original "A" haplotype.

Another way haplotype analysis is useful is that it allows for the extraction of more genetic information when there are missing data or when markers are not fully informative. For example, for marker two, both the "A" and "a" haplotype each have allele 4. Looking at marker two in isolation, it would be impossible to determine whether individuals three, five, and seven inherited the same or different chromosomes from their affected parent, person one, as the marker is not informative. Because marker two is sandwiched between two fully informative markers (markers one and three), however, we know that the segregation pattern, as determined from all the markers taken together, is likely to be correct. (Rarely, two recombinations occur within a short interval, and the possibility of this happening can sometimes complicate haplotype analysis.)

> Haplotype analysis enables adjacent markers to be examined together to interpret how whole chromosomal regions were inherited and recombined within a family.

Linkage disequilibrium

Haplotype analysis can also be used for research purposes to investigate "founder effects" and "linkage disequilibrium."

> Linkage disequilibrium occurs when an allele for a particular gene is distributed in a population by related descent from a common ancestor. Some adjacent genes and/or markers will not yet have had recombination events dissociating them from the allele contributed by the founding individual. Consequently, contemporary individuals in the population who inherit the gene from a common founder will all share a common haplotype in the vicinity of the gene.

For example, from a combination of genealogical data and haplotype analysis, it has been inferred that many American families with Huntington's disease are descended from a common ancestor who apparently resided in Suffolk, England around 1630. Markers that are very closely spaced around the Huntington's disease gene have not yet had a recombination occur between them and the gene. Thus, there is a small chromosomal region that different families, all descended from the same common founder, still have in common.

> Linkage disequilibrium analysis can be used to help positionally clone genes.

In fact, the phenomenon of linkage disequilibrium was used to clone the Huntington's disease gene in the first place, under the assumption that many families not known to be related were descended anyway from a common affected ancestor. The numerous modern families were actually just distant branches of the same original family, whose relationships had long ago become forgotten. Since it was likely that many families came from the same founder, markers from different families that had exactly the same alleles could be used to help infer the narrowest possible region in which the gene must reside.

> Linkage disequilibrium analysis can be used to date the emergence of a particular allele in the population.

For example, a fascinating example of the use of haplotype analysis is the dating of the origin of the CCR5-Δ32 AIDS-resistance allele. CCR5 is a receptor protein present on the surface of macrophages. The Δ32 mutation deletes 32 nucleotides and creates a frame shift that prematurely leads to termination of the altered reading frame. Homozygotes for the Δ32 allele of CCR5 have no obvious illness and, in fact, are quite advantageously resistant to infection by HIV! Chromosomes that have the Δ32 mutation on them all have exactly the same alleles for various markers that flank the CCR5 gene in a small stretch. From this haplotype sharing, it can be deduced that they all must be descended from a common ancestor. From theoretical studies, it can be inferred that the length of the haplotype held in common between these modern day individuals must have taken about 30 or so generations to become "whittled down" to this size. It can be deduced that this mutation first arose about 700 years ago (assuming something like 23 years/generation), and is hypothesized to have coincided with the plague in Europe. It would appear that this mutation was a relatively random event existing in a single individual around the time of the plague and, presumably, became more common in the population because it conferred some degree of resistance to the plague. The plague destroyed much of Europe's population over the next few generations, and the offspring of the individual in which this mutation fortuitously arose enjoyed enormous reproductive success due to the fact that they could survive this epidemic. There is emerging confirmation of this hypothesis. *Yersinia pestis*, the plague bacillus, appears to utilize the CCR5 molecule in order to infect macrophages, a common target of both *Yersinia* and HIV.

We are presently reaching the state where the molecular basis of many, if not most, single gene disorders has been defined. The research enterprise will soon redirect its focus toward common diseases in which the genetic effects will be more difficult to elucidate. Consequently, larger numbers of people will need to be studied and newer methods will require development.

In the future, it is possible that genome-wide screens will be conducted through linkage disequilibrium, rather than the current genetic linkage analysis in place today.

The supposition is that everybody is descended from a small founding population of *homo sapiens* in Africa. Consequently, there was a limited number of original haplotypes corresponding to our common ancestors. Over time, recombination has whittled down the size of any particular haplotype in any particular chromosomal region. In fact, by using the archeological record to estimate the length of time and hence, number of generations that have elapsed since the human species was founded, it is estimated that the length of the common haplotype from the founding human population is about three thousand basepairs. At a small enough scale, then, each of our chromosomes are composites built from chunks of chromosomes originally intact in the very first humans. It should then be possible to identify common haplotypes distributed throughout the genome between any two people. Through the identification of a common haplotype shared by multiple individuals with a particular disease, then, it might be possible to identify chromosomal regions encoding genes responsible for particular illnesses. The advantage of such methods is that since we know that all human beings are ultimately part of the same family, we can just collect people at random (with the disease we are interested in studying) and then set about to identify any regions showing a common haplotype at a frequency significantly greater than chance. Identifying individuals to study should be rather easy; even though hundreds to thousands of cooperating subjects will be required, we will not have to worry about getting their siblings, parents, or other relatives. The hard part lies in the fact that resolving a haplotype to a level less than three thousand basepairs in the human genome (with haploid size of about three billion basepairs) would require looking at about a million markers. And, in a study with about a thousand subjects, then that means "genotyping" about a billion markers. This is not possible using present day microsatellite markers. But, with coming advances in high throughput technology, like DNA chips, it will not be too far in the future when such powerful studies can be used to determine, even the occasionally weak, genetic risk factors underlying all sorts of common and genetically "complex" diseases, such as hypertension, mental illness, diabetes mellitus, and cancer.

· C H A P T E R · 6 ·

DYNAMIC MUTATION

·

- **Fragile X Syndrome**

   Fragile Sites

   The Molecular Basis of Fragile X

   Clinically Observed Patterns of Inheritance

   Summary of Fragile X Inheritance

- **Huntington's Disease**

- **Myotonic Dystrophy**

- **Other Diseases Caused by Unstable Repeats**

· · · · · · · · · · · ·

> **Anticipation:** The clinical observation that an inherited disease displays increasing severity and/or an earlier age of onset (Fig. 6-1) with each subsequent generation.

Anticipation was reported in the early part of the twentieth century for Huntington's disease and another neurodegenerative disorder, myotonic dystrophy,

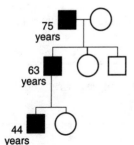

Figure 6-1 Anticipation in the form of a declining age of onset with each generation.

when it was observed that the children of an affected parent were frequently affected at a younger age, or more severely affected, than in the preceding generation. The idea was widely accepted until the late 1940s, when persuasive arguments by a prominent geneticist suggested that anticipation was a statistical artifact that could be attributed to a bias in the way families were ascertained for study. Anticipation was largely forgotten about until the late 1980s. It was then that a series of surprising molecular discoveries, demonstrating that unstable trinucleotide (or "triplet") repeat sequences were the basis of the mutation in Huntington's disease, myotonic dystrophy, and Fragile X syndrome, confirmed anticipation.

FRAGILE X SYNDROME

Fragile X is among the most common causes of mental retardation for both males and females. Affected individuals may also have characteristic dysmorphic features, including a long facies with prominence of the ears, forehead, and jaw. Hyperextensibility of the joints may be seen. Most postpubescent males with fragile X have enlarged testes (macroorchidism). The disease takes its name from the fact that most affected individuals have a "fragile site" demonstrable at the terminus of the long arm of the X chromosome.

FRAGILE SITES

In general, fragile sites are not all that uncommon and are found in many individuals at different chromosomal locations. Fragile sites are chromosomal regions that appear, well, "fragile" when examined microscopically in cells cultured in vitro under particular conditions. The fragile X site, for example, looks like a small bit of the end of the chromosome has broken off and is hanging on thread-like to the rest of the chromosome. The fragile site does not appear in cultured cells from fragile X individuals unless the cells are grown in a media that deprives them of folate and/or thymidine, both metabolites being involved in DNA synthesis. Other fragile sites in the genome may be induced by other similar conditions that impair nucleotide metabolism.

In spite of the name, most fragile sites are not actually places of chromosome breakage—it only just looks that way.

Like most hereditary illnesses resulting from mutation of a gene on the X chromosome, fragile X is inherited as a sex-linked recessive disorder. Males inherit the disease from a carrier mother. The penetrance for females is rather high, however, and results from skewing of X chromosome inactivation in affected females. The inheritance of fragile X, however, is not quite as straightforward as it is for other sex-linked recessive diseases. The likelihood of being affected with fragile X is dependent on the position of the individual in the pedigree. Individuals appearing in a generation subsequent to one in which somebody is already known to have the disease are at a higher risk for having affected children, in accord with anticipation.

THE MOLECULAR BASIS OF FRAGILE X

Fragile X results from mutations in a gene, FMR1, at the location of the fragile site on the X chromosome. The protein product of the gene binds RNA and appears to function in the nuclear export of RNA. The mutation is characteristic and involves "expansion" of a CGG triplet repeat DNA sequence. In normal individuals, there are about 8 to 50 copies of a CGG trinucleotide repeat in the 5' untranslated promoter region of the gene. Individuals with the fragile X syndrome have a mutation comprised of about 200 to 1000 copies of this repetitive trinucleotide sequence. There is a third category of individuals known as "premutation carriers." These individuals are unaffected by fragile X, but are at risk for having children or later descendants with fragile X. They have between about 52 to 200 CGG triplet repeats. Affected individuals with the "full mutation" have greatly reduced transcriptional expression of the fragile X gene (if they are males, who are hemizygous for genes on the X chromosome) or greatly reduced expression from the single allele with the CGG triplet repeat expansion mutation (if they are females, who are heterozygous for genes on the X chromosome, but whose X chromosome genes are also subject to random X inactivation). In the fragile X full mutation, cytosine bases within the repeat tract are methylated. As is the usual case with cytosine methylation in the promoter region of a gene, transcription is switched off, thereby resulting in loss of expression of that allele.

Chromosomes with the fragile X full mutation usually display the fragile site under appropriate culture conditions. The appearance of the fragile site is evidently a direct result of the unusually long GC basepair enriched sequence. There are extremely rare individuals who have the fragile X syndrome resulting not from expansion of CGG repeats, but rather, as a result of an inactivating point mutation in the coding sequence of the gene.

Genetic testing is available for the fragile X syndrome and has replaced the much less sensitive and older approach based on cell culture to demonstrate the fragile site on the X chromosome. The test consists of a Southern blot probed with a fragment of the fragile X gene to directly detect expansions of the CGG repeat in the promoter region. As a secondary confirmation, the methylation status of the repeat is also usually checked with a pair of restriction enzymes that differentially recognize methylated cytosine residues.

CLINICALLY OBSERVED PATTERNS OF INHERITANCE

Although complicated, the genetics of the fragile X syndrome can be methodically explained. The important concept to appreciate is that once triplet repeat sequences have expanded to a certain length, they become unstable during meiosis and are at risk of expanding to an even greater length with a meiosis in each subsequent generation in the family. There is some threshold number of repeats that, once crossed, turns a premutation into a full mutation capable of causing the disease.

Expansion of the fragile X CGG triplet repeat from a normal length (approximately 8 to 50 copies of the triplet repeat) to the premutation length (about 52 to 200 repeats) almost never happens. From haplotype analysis and linkage disequilibrium studies of chromosomes containing a fragile X premutation or full mutation, it has been determined that this event has happened only rarely in human history, since many of the premutations and full mutations appear to have been inherited from a remote, common founder.

On the other hand, expansion of a premutation sized repeat to a full mutation (about 200 to 1000 triplet repeats) is rather common, but it can only occur through a female meiosis. The precise risk that a premutation will expand to a full mutation is dependent on the length of the premutation repeat in the heterozygous female carrier. The greater the length of the premutation, the more likely it is to expand in a female meiosis. In general, for most situations, we can assume that there is an 80% probability that a female premutation repeat will expand to a full mutation length during meiosis. However, when the premutation repeat length reaches 90 or more triplets, then expansion to a full mutation happens with near certainty.

The penetrance of fragile X in males with the full mutation is 100%. In females with the full mutation, the penetrance is about 30 to 50% (as a result of skewed Lyonization). Finally, the sperm of males with the fragile X syndrome appears to contain only X chromosomes with the premutation. This means that in the rare situations where a mentally retarded male with the fragile X syndrome could father a daughter, the daughter will inherit only the premutation and will not be affected. (Male children of an affected male will not inherit the father's X chromosome and, therefore, have no risk of being affected.)

SUMMARY OF FRAGILE X INHERITANCE

- Normal   < 52 CGG repeats
  Premutation   ~ 52–200 CGG repeats
  Full mutation   > 200 CGG repeats
- Expansion from normal to premutation virtually never occurs.
- Expansion from premutation to full mutation only occurs through female meiosis.
- Expansion from premutation to full mutation is dependent on the length of the premutation repeat, but, in general, there is about an 80% probability of this happening during a female meiosis for repeats less than 90 triplets and 100% probability when there are 90 or more triplet repeats.
- One-hundred percent penetrance in males with the full mutation. About 30 to 50% penetrance in females with the full mutation.

Let us work through the following examples to illustrate the inheritance of the fragile X syndrome. Each small pedigree represents each of the ten possible combinations of situations involving a parent of either sex with either a premutation or a full mutation with a pending pregnancy with the fetus of either sex. (The symbols for clinically affected individuals are blackened, as is the usual custom. Carriers of the premutation are denoted with a small dot in the middle of their pedigree symbol. And for the sake of convenience, we will use a non-standard nomenclature in which women who are clinically unaffected carriers of the full mutation will be denoted with a circular pedigree symbol with a large dot in the middle.)

In the first case, the father is known to be a premutation carrier, who therefore is clinically unaffected. The mother is known to have two normal length repeats in each of her X chromosomes. The fetus is known by ultrasound to be female (Fig. 6-2). (Ultrasound is pretty good, but is usually not relied on completely

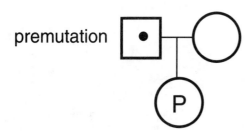

premutation

Figure 6-2   Premutation father and female fetus.

for fetal sex determination, but we are doing so here for didactic purposes solely to illustrate the genetic transmission of fragile X.) Since the fetus is female, we know that it obligatorily inherited the father's X chromosome, which has the pre-mutation. The premutation does not have the possibility of expanding to a full mutation during paternal meiosis, so the fetus will inherit a premutation. The fetus, therefore, has no chance of manifesting the fragile X syndrome; however, she will be a premutation carrier.

The next two examples consider the case of a pregnant woman known to be a carrier of the fragile X premutation (i.e., the fetus from the case before has now grown up).

If the fetus is male (Fig. 6-3), there is a 50% probability that the X chromo-some with the premutation will segregate to the oocyte during maternal meiosis, just as there is with standard sex-linked recessive disorders. However, we also must consider the additional possibility that the CGG triplet repeat will expand in length during the maternal meiosis from the premutation range to the full muta-tion range. This probability is actually dependent on the exact length of the mater-nal premutation (the larger it is, the higher the probability of expansion), but in most clinical situations, it is reasonable to assume that the probability of this hap-pening is 80%. Thus, there is a 50% chance that the male fetus will not inherit the chromosome containing the abnormal CGG repeat from his mother and will be neither clinically affected nor a carrier of the premutation. If the fetus does inherit the chromosome with the abnormal CGG repeat (50% probability), there is an 80% probability of it expanding to the full mutation; therefore, there is a 50% × 80% = 40% probability that the fetus will have the full mutation and be affected with the fragile X syndrome. Conversely, if the fetus does inherit the abnormal maternal X chromosome (50% probability), there is also a 20% probability that the repeat will not expand to full mutation length; thus, there is a 50% × 20% = 10% probability that the fetus will inherit a fragile X premutation and be clini-cally unaffected (i.e., that the outcome would produce the father of the previous example). Reassuringly, the sum of the probabilities of all possible outcomes is 1.

How do things change if the fetus is female (Fig. 6-4)? The only thing that is different is that the completely normal father has contributed his X chromo-

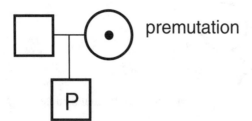

premutation

Figure 6-3   Premutation mother and male fetus.

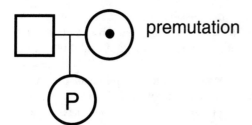

premutation

Figure 6-4   Premutation mother
and female fetus.

some to the fetus, rather than his Y chromosome, to make the fetus female. So, everything works identically to the previous example, but with the additional consideration of sex-dependent penetrance of the fragile X phenotype in females. There is still a 50% probability of the fetus inheriting the X chromosome with the abnormal length CGG repeat from the mother, just as there is with standard sex-linked recessive inheritance. There is also still an 80% probability that the pre-mutation length CGG repeat will expand to the full mutation during the maternal meiosis. The outcomes are then as follows. There is a 50% probability that the fetus will inherit the mother's normal X chromosome and will be both unaffected and a non-carrier. There is a 50% probability that the fetus will inherit the mother's abnormal X chromosome times a 20% probability that the premutation will not expand resulting in a 50% × 20% = 10% probability that the fetus will carry the fragile X premutation but will be clinically unaffected. The premutation will expand about 80% of the time, however; so, there is also a 50% × 80% = 40% probability that the fetus will inherit the full mutation. Since the penetrance of the fragile X full mutation in heterozygous females is about 50%, there is a 50% × 40% = 20% probability that the fetus will be clinically affected with the fragile X syndrome and, of course, a 50% × 40% = 20% probability that the fetus will have the full mutation but turn out to be unaffected with the fragile X syndrome.

We now move on to pregnancies involving individuals produced by the above situation.

In the next example (Fig. 6-5), we have a male with the premutation whose normal mate is expecting a male fetus. Just as with standard sex-linked recessive

premutation

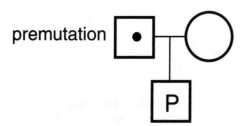

Figure 6-5   Premutation father
and male fetus.

inheritance, there is no male-to-male transmission because a son only inherits the Y chromosome from the father. Therefore, there is a zero probability that the fetus will inherit the premutation from his father and a zero probability that the fetus will have the fragile X syndrome.

Rarely, males with the fragile X syndrome father children of their own. (Mental retardation greatly reduces male fitness, but the sad fact is that the converse may not be true. Mental retardation in females may increase fitness by making them more vulnerable to nonconsensual sexual relations.) What happens when a male with the fragile X syndrome (and consequently, the full mutation) fathers a male child (Fig. 6-6)? Of course, just as before, there is no male-to-male transmission of the X chromosome, so the fetus will inherit neither the pre- or full mutation and has no chance of being affected. A strange thing happens, however, in the rare circumstance where a male with the fragile X syndrome should father a female conception (Fig. 6-7). Just as with ordinary sex-linked recessive inheritance, the daughter will necessarily inherit the father's solitary X chromosome. We should expect, therefore, that the daughter will have the full mutation and be at 50% risk for penetrance of having the syndrome. Strangely enough, the sperm from a male with the full mutation and the fragile X syndrome appears to only contain premutation length repeats. Therefore, daughters of an affected male have zero chance to be clinically affected, but will necesssarily be carriers of the premutation.

Let us continue with pregnancies involving women with the full mutation. In the first case (Fig. 6-8), a clinically unaffected woman hemizygous for the full

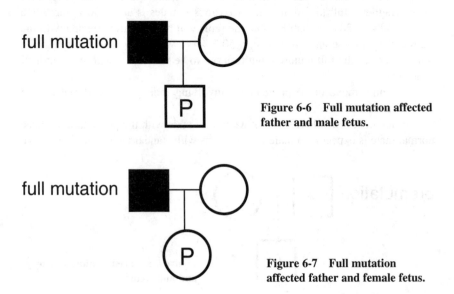

full mutation

P

Figure 6-6   Full mutation affected father and male fetus.

full mutation

P

Figure 6-7   Full mutation affected father and female fetus.

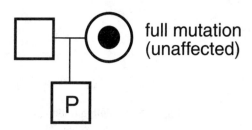

full mutation
(unaffected)

Figure 6-8   Full mutation non-penetrant mother and male fetus.

mutation is expecting a male fetus. Just as with regular sex-linked recessive inheritance, there is a 50% probability that the fetus will inherit the abnormal maternal X chromosome. Since the X chromosome already has the full mutation, there is a 50% probability that the male fetus will inherit the full mutation and be clinically affected. Conversely, there is a 50% probability that he will not inherit the abnormal X chromosome from his mother and will neither be affected nor a premutation carrier.

Compared to the previous example, what is different when a clinically affected woman hemizygous for the full mutation is expecting a male fetus (Fig. 6-9)? Nothing. There is a 50% probability that the male fetus will inherit the maternal X chromosome containing the fragile X full mutation, and therefore, be clinically affected, and a 50% probability that the fetus will inherit the normal X chromosome (and, of course, be unaffected).

Last, we must consider the effect of sex limited penetrance when a woman hemizygous for the fragile X full mutation is expecting a female child (Figs. 6-10 and 6-11). Just as before, it does not matter whether the woman is penetrant

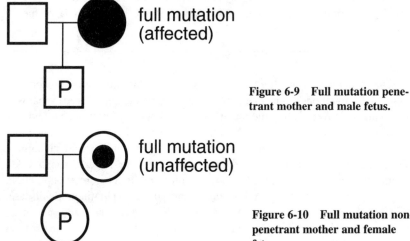

full mutation
(affected)

Figure 6-9   Full mutation penetrant mother and male fetus.

full mutation
(unaffected)

Figure 6-10   Full mutation non-penetrant mother and female fetus.

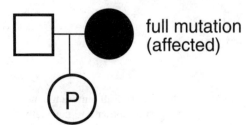

full mutation
(affected)

Figure 6-11   Full mutation penetrant mother and female fetus.

(i.e., clinically affected) with the fragile X syndrome. There is a 50% probability that she will transmit the abnormal chromosome with the full mutation and a 50% probability that she will transmit the normal chromosome. So, 50% of the time her daughters will be clinically unaffected and have neither the pre- nor full mutation. The other 50% of the time that the full mutation is inherited from a mother hemizygous for the full mutation, there is a 50% probability of penetrance. Thus, there is a 50% × 50% = 25% probability of having a clinically unaffected daughter with the full mutation and a 50% × 50% = 25% probability of having a clinically affected daughter with the full mutation.

HUNTINGTON'S DISEASE

Huntington's disease is an autosomal dominant, adult-onset, severe neurodegenerative disorder characterized in the initial stages by mild cognitive symptoms with progressive choreiform (involuntary dance-like) movement disorder. Psychiatric disorders may also occur. At the anatomic level, there is degeneration of the caudate and putamen in the basal ganglia of the brain.

The responsible gene, huntingtin, is expressed ubiquitously throughout the brain and the function of the gene product still remains undetermined. What was a surprising discovery is that the mutation in every individual with Huntington's disease is an expansion of the DNA triplet repeat sequence CAG, contained in a protein coding sequence of the gene, and encoding the amino acid glutamine. Individuals without Huntington's disease normally have fewer than 35 CAG repeats, although the repeat length is polymorphic among the normal population. Individuals with 40 or more CAG repeats usually develop Huntington's disease, while people with 36 to 39 may not develop the disease or, if so, only at an advanced age. The huntingtin protein from individuals with a CAG repeat tract expansion will then have an elongated tract encoding polyglutamine within the polypeptide.

The age of onset of the disease can be largely explained by the number of repeats an individual has (Fig. 6-12), the greater the number of repeats, the earlier the age of onset. Just as with the fragile X syndrome, once the number of repeats passes a critical threshold, the repeat tract becomes unstable and is at risk for further increases in length with every subsequent meiosis. Anticipation is thus explained by the CAG repeat length increasing from one generation to the next.

For most trinucleotide repeat genes, there is a strong inverse correlation between the length of the repeat and the age of onset or severity of the disease, thus, offering a molecular genetic explanation for anticipation.

There are similarities and differences between the repeat instability in Huntington's disease compared to fragile X syndrome. The premutation category of repeat length is in the range of 27 to 36 CAG repeats, although expansion into a full mutation range is infrequent. A difference is that, unlike the case for fragile X syndrome, meiotic repeat expansion, especially large expansions, occurs preferentially during *paternal* meiosis. Alleles inherited from mothers usually have a repeat length that remains the same or expands or contracts by just a few CAG triplets. Rarely, the repeat may reach a length of 65 or more. In these extraordinary circumstances, the disease will have an onset during childhood.

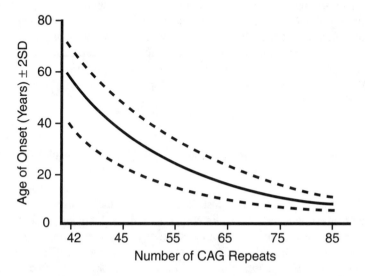

Figure 6-12   Inverse relationship between triplet repeat length and age of onset in Huntington's disease.

> Length expansion usually occurs preferentially through one parental sex for each of the different trinucleotide repeat disease genes.

Presymptomatic diagnostic testing for Huntington's disease is simple and consists of a PCR assay to determine the length of the CAG repeat tract. Ethical issues relating to the use of the test are not so simple, however. It is recommended that individuals at risk for inheriting Huntington's disease who undergo molecular genetic testing for presymptomatic diagnosis, receive appropriate pre-test genetic counseling and post-test psychological support.

MYOTONIC DYSTROPHY

Myotonic dystrophy (also known as dystrophia myotonica and commonly abbreviated "DM") is an autosomal dominantly inherited syndrome whose principal feature is "myotonia." Myotonia is an inability of a muscle to relax following contraction. In individuals with DM, the handshake typically will be prolonged. When myotonia is severe, if the patient is asked to make a fist and then release it, he or she may need to use the contralateral hand to unfold the fingers. Another feature of DM is myopathic weakness. This is most prominent in the facial musculature, and there is a characteristic myopathic facies with a tendency toward bilateral ptosis of the eyelids and an open mouth. There may additionally be cardiac involvement; individuals with DM are at risk for cardiac arrhythmia, most often relatively benign first-degree heart block, but occasionally, they have malignant ventricular tachyarrhythmias that predispose to sudden cardiac death. Cardiomyopathy is also a common feature. Two other prominent features of DM include the early onset of an unusual appearing cataract (described as a Christmas tree) and a predisposition to diabetes mellitus.

The mutation responsible for myotonic dystrophy is also a pathologic expansion of a trinucleotide repeat sequence, in this case CTG located in the 3′ untranslated region of a protein kinase gene expressed in muscle. (Remember that CTG is really the same as CAG; it is just the sequence of the complementary strand running in the opposite 3′ to 5′ direction. But unlike Huntington's disease, the CTG repeat expansion in DM is not translated into a protein coding sequence.) It is unknown how the expanded CTG repeat sequence interferes with expression of the protein kinase gene, in whose 3′ untranslated region it is located. There is some evidence that the transcript from the pathologic allele fails to get exported from the nucleus to the cytoplasm, therefore, does not get translated, and results in reduced levels of expression of the protein. There is also good evidence that some of the related features of DM, like diabetes mellitus and a predisposition to other disorders of endocrine function, may result from the expanded repeat having an influence on the transcriptional expression of neighboring genes.

DM, like the rest of this group of diseases caused by unstable triplet repeat expansions, demonstrates anticipation. In general, just as for Huntington's disease, there is an inverse correlation between the age of onset of disease and length of the repeat tract; and a direct relationship between the severity of symptoms and the length of the repeat tract. Just like the other diseases, meiotic expansion of the repeated sequence occurs preferentially in the meiosis of just one sex, in this case the mother. In normal individuals, there are typically fewer than 5 to 35 CTG triplet repeats. Individuals with 50 to 100 repeats may have milder expression of the disease. As the repeat length increases, the disease becomes progressively more severe with a much earlier age of onset.

Unlike the other triplet repeat diseases, there is occasionally massive expansion of the repeat in a maternal meiosis. Rather than a step-wise progression of repeat length occurring over several generations, a mildly affected woman with relatively few repeats may give birth to a child with several hundred or thousand repeats. In this case, the onset of the disease is evident at birth, and the disease is known as "congenital" myotonic dystrophy. Disease manifestations are severe and are characterized by generalized hypotonia, respiratory and feeding difficulty in neonates, and often, mental retardation should the child survive infancy.

Occasionally the CTG repeat tract will be observed to contract in length between generations. This appears to occur exclusively in male meiosis.

OTHER DISEASES CAUSED BY UNSTABLE REPEATS

There are other inherited diseases caused by expansions of unstable triplet repeats, and the location of the repeat in their respective gene is indicated in Figure 6-13.

Spinal cerebellar ataxia is a genetically heterogeneous autosomal dominantly inherited disease characterized by the adult onset of progressive ataxia (poorly coordinated movement) with accompanying degenerative changes in the cerebellum and brainstem. Some forms of the disease may also be associated with cognitive changes, retinopathy with blindness, and sensorimotor peripheral neuropathy. Anticipation in the inheritance of the spinal cerebellar ataxias has been observed. A number of different loci for spinal cerebellar ataxia have now been mapped, and many of the genes have been cloned. The responsible mutation in every family and for every gene is, just like with Huntington's disease, an

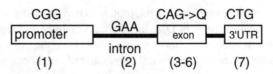

(1) fragile X syndrome
(2) Friedreich's ataxia
(3) Huntington's disease
(4) spinal cerebellar ataxia
(5) spinal bulbar muscular atrophy
(6) dentatorubral-pallidoluysian atrophy
(7) myotonic dystrophy

Figure 6-13 Location of the repeat in the gene for some diseases caused by unstable triplet repeats.

expanded polyglutamine-encoding CAG tract within a protein coding sequence in an exon.

Friedreich's ataxia is unique in that it is both the only disease caused by dynamic mutation in which the repeat is a GAA sequence and the only disease in which the repeat is located in the intron of the gene.

Huntington's disease, spinal cerebellar ataxia, and several other inherited neurodegenerative diseases result from expansion of a CAG triplet repeat encoding polyglutamine. Fragile X results from expansion and hypermethylation of a CGG repeat in the 5′ in the promoter of the responsible gene, leading to loss of expression of the gene. The CTG repeat responsible for myotonic dystrophy is contained within the 3′ untranslated region of a protein kinase and the pathogenesis of the disease is still unknown.

· C H A P T E R · 7 ·

CYTOGENETICS

·

· · · · · · · · · · · · ·

Cytogenetics refers to the study of chromosomes, their structure, and their inheritance. Why should we be concerned about chromosomal abnormalities? The answer is because they are common:

Of all newborns, about 1 in 150 have a chromosome abnormality. At least 50% of first trimester spontaneous abortions have a chromosome abnormality. Approximately 2% of all pregnancies in women over 35 years old have a chromosomal abnormality. Acquired chromosomal abnormalities are a common feature of malignancies, especially of leukemia and other hematopoietic cancer.

Constitutional cytogenetic abnormality: Chromosome make-up at birth and may be inherited.
Acquired cytogenetic abnormality: Typically not present at birth, limited to certain tissues, and not inherited.

In any discussion of cytogenetics, it is important to first distinguish between "constitutional" and "acquired" chromosomal abnormalities. Constitutional refers to the genetic make-up at birth. These abnormalities are usually present in every cell of the body, are often inherited, and are at risk of being transmitted to children. Acquired chromosomal abnormalities usually occur after birth (or at least after conception), are in a limited distribution of the cells of the body (often times just in a tumor, for example), are not inherited, and are not at risk for being transmitted to future generations.

CYTOGENETIC ORGANIZATION OF THE HUMAN GENOME

The diploid human genome consists of 6 to 7 billion base pairs of DNA organized into 23 pairs of chromosomes. Each chromosome consists of a single continuous strand of DNA complexed with histone and other proteins. This combination of DNA and protein is arranged in structures of progressively greater degrees of organization. The double helix is wound into a nucleosome fiber, that in turn is coiled into a solenoid, then assembled into chromatin, and finally the chromatid.

CHROMOSOME ANALYSIS AND CLASSIFICATION

To analyze chromosomes, they need to be prepared from cells that are actively dividing. Peripheral blood leukocytes are most often used for routine chromosome analysis because of the ease of obtaining the specimen. Other tissues used for chromosome analysis include bone marrow samples (used mainly for the diagnosis of hematologic malignancies), solid tumors, skin (used frequently to detect mosaicism), and amniotic fluid cells and chorionic villi for prenatal diagnosis of chromosomal disorders.

Before chromosomal banding techniques were developed in the early 1970s, cytogeneticists classified the chromosomes into different groups on the basis of centromere position and chromosome size. The centromere is a standard cytological landmark that divides the chromosome into two arms—p (for petite), or short arm, and q for the long arm. Human chromosomes are classified by centromere position into three types—metacentric (arms of approximately equal length), submetacentric (arms of unequal length), and acrocentric (centromere near one end of the chromosome) (Fig. 7-1). The p arm of the acrocentric

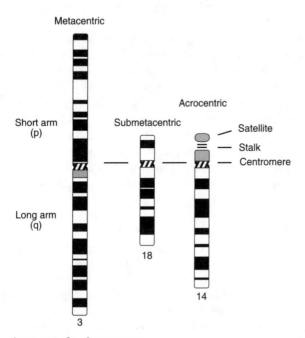

Figure 7-1   Anatomy of a chromosome.

chromosome is composed of a satellite and stalk region that contains redundant copies of ribosomal RNA genes.

In addition, the chromosomes are arranged according to size, from largest to smallest, with one exception—the sex chromosomes are always placed in the lower right-hand corner. This ordered configuration of chromosomes is called a karyotype.

Karyotype: Array of photographs of chromosomes ordered according to their length and the relative position of their centromeres.

The development of different staining methods in the early 1970s revolutionized cytogenetics, because individual identification of each chromosome became possible. Each chromosome has a characteristic banding pattern, enabling the cytogeneticist to distinguish one chromosome from the other and more accurately arrange the karyotype. The following are staining techniques used in cytogenetics laboratories.

1. **G banding.** The G stands for "giemsa," which is the dye most often used to visualize the bands. This is the most widely used staining method in the United States.
2. **R banding.** The name R banding is derived from "reverse-banding" because the light and dark bands are the reverse of G bands. This technique is often helpful in studying the ends of chromosomes, as in the case of distal deletions or rearrangements.
3. **Q banding.** This was the first staining method developed and stands for quinacrine banding. Quinacrine is a fluorescent stain that requires the use of a fluorescent microscope and thus, is not readily used today in the United States. Bright Q bands are comparable to dark G bands.
4. **NOR (nucleolar organizing region) staining.** This technique stains the ribosomal RNA genes located near the stalk and satellite region of the acrocentric chromosomes.

There appears to be a correlation between the structural and functional organization of the chromosomes. For example, there are different characteristics of G-light bands versus G-dark bands (Table 7-1). G-light bands have a higher GC content and are early replicating in the S phase of the cell cycle. Most importantly, G-light bands are thought to contain the most genes (both housekeeping and tissue-specific genes). In contrast, G-dark bands have a higher A-T content, replicate late in S phase, and contain fewer genes. Therefore, it is thought that chromosomal abnormalities involving "gene-rich" G-light bands may have more clinical significance than those involving "gene-poor" G-dark bands.

TABLE 7-1
DARK VERSUS LIGHT BANDS

G-LIGHT BANDS	G-DARK BANDS
GC-rich DNA	AT-rich DNA
Early replicating	Late replicating
Many genes	Few genes

The cytogeneticist can obtain various levels of banding based on the quality and origin of the chromosome preparation. Typically, the higher the band level, the better the resolution. Generally speaking, bone marrow samples will have a resolution at the 350 band level, whereas amniotic fluid is usually at the 450 to 550 band level. A routine blood study at our institution implies that there is a 550 to 750 band level, and prometaphase blood study implies that there is a 750 to 850 band level. The band level is an important factor when determining whether a chromosome analysis should be repeated. Subtle rearrangements may not be detected at the 450 band level but may be visualized at the 750 band level.

> The band level is an important factor in determining the quality of the chromosome analysis. A higher band level implies a more informative study.

A drawing of the human karyotype, illustrated in Figure 7-2, is referred to as an ideogram. Notice that the G bands have been numbered with a standardized system, which allows one to define structural and numerical abnormalities. Each arm is first divided into regions (first number) and then each region into specific bands (second number). Numbering is from the centromere outward on each arm, the region number and, finally, the band number. For example, band 2p21 (pronounced "two-pee-two-one," not "two-pee-twenty-one") indicates chromosome 2, short arm, region 2 band 1.

Every physician should know some basic principles of cytogenetic nomenclature. A standardized system of karyotype nomenclature has been defined. The system of notation is as follows: first indicate the total number of chromosomes, followed by a comma, and then by the chromosome constitution. For example, 46, XX for female and 46, XY for male. If an abnormality is present, it is described using specific notations. For example, 47, XY, +21 (male with trisomy 21 Down syndrome). Examples of standard nomenclature for some chromosome abnormalities are listed in Table 7-2.

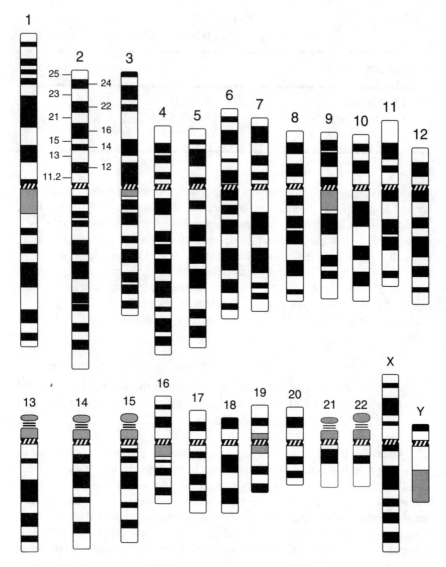

Figure 7-2   400 band resolution, G-banded ideogram. © David Adler, 1995.

TABLE 7-2
STANDARD NOMENCLATURE FOR CHROMOSOME KARYOTYPES

KARYOTYPE	DESCRIPTION
46,XX	Normal female
47,XY,+21	Male with trisomy 21 (Down syndrome)
47,XX,+21/46,XX	Female who is a mosaic of trisomy 21 cells and normal cells
46,XX,del(6)(p25)	Female with deletion of the short arm of chromosome 6 band 25
46,XY,dup(4p)	Male with a duplication of the short arm of chromosome 4
45,XX,der(14;21)(q10;q10)	Female with balanced Robertsonian translocation of chromosome 21 and 14; one normal 21 and one normal 14 are missing; this woman has greater risk for a child with Down syndrome
46,XX,t(4;5)(p13;q22)	Female with balanced reciprocal translocation between chromosomes 4 and 5; the break points are at 4p13 and 5q22
46,XY,inv(2)(p21q23)	Male with a pericentric inversion on chromosome 2 from p21 to q23
46,X,i(Xp)	Female with one normal X chromosome and an isochromosome of the short arm of the X chromosome

MOLECULAR CYTOGENETICS

Routine and high resolution chromosome analysis permit the detection of numerical and structural chromosome abnormalities, but only to the extent to which we can actually see these changes under the microscope. Small chromosomal deletions, translocations, and marker chromosomes are difficult and sometimes, impossible, to identify with routine analysis. With the introduction of fluorescence in situ hybridization (FISH) in the early 1990s, we are now able to simultaneously assess molecular and cytologic information.

FISH analysis has revolutionized the field of cytogenetics by allowing for the identification of small deletions, translocations, and other chromosomal rearrangements too small to be detectable by ordinary karyotype staining.

FISH is a technique in which a labeled chromosome-specific DNA segment (probe) is hybridized with metaphase, prophase, or interphase chromosomes and then visualized under a fluorescence microscope. Several types of FISH probes are available depending on the particular application in question.

1. **Alphoid repeats.** Centromere repeat sequences that are chromosome-specific. They produce very intense, tight signals that are easy to count in interphase nuclei.
2. **Whole chromosome paint (WCP).** A technique used to paint the entire chromosome of interest. WCPs are useful in the detection of such chromosomal rearrangements as unbalanced translocations and marker chromosomes. The paints are derived by amplifying and labeling by PCR individual chromosomes that have been isolated by flow cytometry.
3. **Sequence specific probes.** Perhaps the most frequently used FISH probes in the diagnostic setting. This type of probe enables one to target a critical deletion region that is responsible for a specific syndrome. Some of the more common microdeletion syndrome for which FISH probes are available are indicated in Table 7-3.
4. **Spectral karyotyping.** A recent advancement in molecular cytogenetics, which refers to complete chromosome karyotyping by FISH, using multiple

TABLE 7-3
MICRODELETION SYNDROMES

SYNDROME	CLINICAL FEATURES	CHROMOSOMAL DELETION
Prader-Willi	Mental retardation, short stature, obesity, hypotonia, characteristic facies, small hands and feet	15q11-13
Smith-Magenis	Mental retardation, dysmorphic features, unique behavioral features	17p11.2
Velocardiofacial	Learning disability/mental retardation, cleft palate, congenital heart defect, characteristic facies, predisposition to mental illness	22q11.2
Williams	Mild mental retardation, characteristic facies, aortic stenosis, unique personality of overfriendliness and possible exceptional musical talents	7q11

fluorochromes. Each of the 23 pairs of chromosomes can be distinguished with a different color. Spectral karyotyping is useful in characterizing complex chromosomal abnormalities.

CHROMOSOMAL ABNORMALITIES

Chromosomal abnormalities may be divided into two broad categories— numerical and structural abnormalities. Numerical abnormalities are simply abnormalities of chromosome number (i.e., polyploidy and aneuploidy). Structural abnormalities include chromosomal rearrangements, deletions, and duplications.

NUMERICAL ABNORMALITIES

Numerical abnormalities consist of those due to extra or missing chromosomes (aneuploidy) as well as multiples of the haploid chromosome number (polyploidy). Aneuploidy may involve either autosomes or sex chromosomes. Most common are monosomies (45 chromosomes) and trisomies (47 chromosomes).

Most aneuploid conditions are the result of nondisjunction, the failure of chromosomes to disjoin during meiosis (Fig. 7-3). At the top of Figure 7-3, each

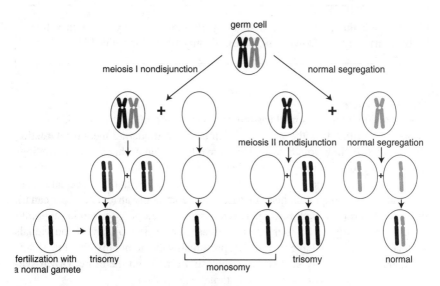

Figure 7-3 Nondisjunction leading to aneuploidy.

parental homolog of the same chromosome is depicted in a synaptic complex. Note that nondisjunction can occur at either meiosis I or meiosis II. When it occurs at meiosis I (left side of the figure), both parental homologs are included in the first division products, but they then segregate normally, except for the fact that there are two copies of one chromosome. Conversely (right side of figure), meiosis I can proceed normally, followed by nondisjunction in meiosis II. When that happens, two copies of the same parental homolog segregate into the gamete. In either case, however, following fertilization with a gamete containing a normal chromosome complement, the resulting zygote will either be trisomic or monosomic for the chromosome that did not disjoin. For simplicity, we are ignoring the impact of recombination in the nondisjunction process. In reality, the effect of recombination allows the investigator to determine whether the nondisjunction occurred in meiosis I or meiosis II. From such studies, it has been found that the overwhelming majority of cases of nondisjunction occur during meiosis I of maternal gametogenesis.

Most autosomal aneuploidy is the result of maternal meiosis I nondisjunction, which is associated with advanced maternal age.

Autosomal aneuploidy

There are three survivable trisomy syndromes that may result in a live birth, trisomy 21 (Down syndrome), trisomy 18, and trisomy 13.

Down syndrome
The most common autosomal trisomy is Down syndrome, with an incidence of 1 in 800 live births. It is the most common cause of moderate mental retardation (IQ 40 to 60). Individuals with Down syndrome have characteristic findings including hypotonia, unique facial features (flat nasal bridge, upslanting palpebral fissures, epicanthal folds, Brushfield spots of the iris, flat midface, and small dysplastic ears), congenital heart disease (most commonly atrioventricular canal), duodenal atresia, as well as an increased risk of developing leukemia, hypothyroidism, and early onset Alzheimer's disease. The vast majority of individuals with Down syndrome have trisomy 21, presumably due to nondisjunction. Maternal nondisjunction is typical (usually meiosis I error) and therefore, Down syndrome is associated with advanced maternal age (AMA).

> The recurrence risk for parents with a child with trisomy 21 to have an additional child with an autosomal trisomy is approximately 1% or the maternal age-related risk, whichever is greater.

In a minority of cases (approximately 2% to 4%), Down syndrome is the result of a Robertsonian translocation. In other words, one parent is a Robertsonian translocation carrier (possesses a balanced translocation between two acrocentric chromosomes), which predisposes to offspring with an unbalanced chromosome complement. The chromosomes may segregate abnormally in the offspring of a Robertsonian translocation carrier (Fig. 7-4). Note that during meiosis, the two normal chromosomes pair with the translocation chromosome in an unusual "triradial" synapse. There are three different ways that the triradial synapse may be resolved, one "alternate" segregation, and two different and perpendicular "adjacent" segregations. Notice that the gametes produced by alternate (balanced) segregation have the normal amount of genetic material and

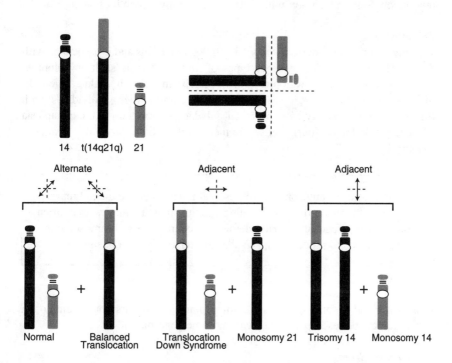

Figure 7-4   Synapse formation and segregation of a Robertsonian translocation chromosome.

would lead to a normal phenotype, when fertilized by a normal gamete. Those gametes produced by either adjacent (unbalanced) segregation have either too much or too little genetic material and after fertilization, would yield an abnormal trisomic or monosomic phenotype, respectively. Only the first three possibilities are viable, whereas monosomy 21, trisomy 14, and monosomy 14 rarely would survive to full term. Although the first three conceptions are compatible with survival, they are not seen in equal frequency, presumably due to prenatal loss. The empirically observed recurrence risk for a Robertsonian translocation mother is 10% to 15%, whereas in the father it is 1% to 2%. Therefore, it is important to always obtain a karyotype on a child with a clinical diagnosis of Down syndrome.

Trisomy 18
Trisomy 18 is a less common trisomy (approximately 1 in 6000 live births). It is also due to maternal nondisjunction and associated with AMA. Clinical findings include prenatal growth retardation, characteristic facial features, (small ears, small mouth, and micrognathia), congenital heart disease, and severe mental retardation. Survival is poor, with a 50% mortality by 1 month of age.

Trisomy 13
Trisomy 13 occurs in approximately 1 in 10,000 live births and is associated with AMA. These babies have various types of midline defects such as holoprosencephaly (incomplete development of the forebrain), cleft lip/palate, microphthalmia, congenital heart disease, and renal abnormalities. Individuals with trisomy 13 also typically have postaxial polydactyly (extra digits), cutis aplasia (skin defect on the occiput), and severe mental retardation. Survival is similar to trisomy 18.

Characteristics of autosomal chromosomal imbalances are mental retardation, growth retardation, and multiple congenital anomalies that often result in early fetal or neonatal demise. In contrast, sex chromosome aneuploidy tends to produce a survivable and relatively mild phenotype.

Sex chromosome aneuploidy
Monosomy and trisomy of the sex chromosomes also occurs not uncommonly. The following are examples of sex chromosome abnormalities.

Turner's syndrome
The incidence of Turner's syndrome is approximately 1 in 5000 live female births. However, the overall incidence is much higher as the majority of conceptions are lost prenatally. Girls with Turner's syndrome have many features in

common including short stature, edema of hands/feet at birth, webbed neck, broad chest with widely spaced nipples, cubitus valgus (widened carrying angle of the arms), congenital heart disease (coarctation of aorta most common), kidney abnormalities and gonadal dysgenesis resulting in a lack of secondary sex characteristics, and amenorrhea and infertility in the vast majority of females. These girls require ovarian hormone replacement therapy and may receive growth hormone with equivocal results. These females have normal intelligence but many have difficulties with spatial perception. Approximately 50% of individuals with Turner's syndrome have a 45, X genotype as the result of paternal nondisjunction (meiotic error in the father), whereas 30% to 40% of individuals are mosaic for the 45, X cell line and another cell line (most commonly 46, XX). Females with 45, X / 46, XY mosaicism are at an increased risk of gonadoblastoma and should have their gonads (present in an underdeveloped, "streak" form) removed. The remaining 10% to 20% of individuals with Turner's syndrome have a structural X chromosome abnormality such as an X isochromosome (abnormally symmetric X chromosome comprised of either two p arms or two q arms reflected about the centromere) or a deletion of the short or long arm of one X chromosome.

Klinefelter's syndrome
Males with Klinefelter's syndrome have an additional X chromosome represented as 47, XXY. The incidence of this sex chromosome abnormality is 1 in 1000 live male births and is, therefore, quite common. These males tend to have tall stature, a euchanoid (female-like) body habitus, gynecomastia (with an increased risk of breast cancer), and testicular atrophy (characterized by a lack of secondary sex characteristics and infertility). These men typically do not have mental retardation but may have a lower IQ compared to their siblings. The extra X chromosome is maternal in origin in the majority of cases, and, therefore, there is an increased incidence of Klinefelter's syndrome with AMA.

47, XXX females
The incidence of 47, XXX females is approximately 1 in 1000 live female births. Most cases are the result of maternal nondisjunction, and, thus, there is an increased risk of 47, XXX females with AMA. These women are often tall for their families and may have a slight reduction in IQ compared to their siblings. Fertility is typically normal.

47, XYY males
This sex chromosome abnormality is also quite common with an incidence of 1 in 1000 live male births. These males may be taller than average but otherwise have a normal phenotype. Fertility is normal. IQ may be slightly below that of their siblings. Contrary to what was once thought, 47, XYY males are not more inclined to commit violent crimes. However, behavior problems such as attention

deficit hyperactivity disorder may be more common. Note that this chromosome abnormality is not the result of maternal nondisjunction (how could it be with an extra Y chromosome?), and, therefore, there is not an increased incidence with AMA.

Polysomy
Polysomy for sex chromosomes (i.e., 49, XXXXX) has been reported, and it appears that the incidence of mental retardation and physical abnormalities increases with an increasing number of sex chromosomes.

STRUCTURAL ABNORMALITIES
Structural chromosome abnormalities may be balanced or unbalanced. Balanced rearrangements do not produce a loss or gain of chromosome material and usually cause no phenotypic effect. Individuals with a balanced rearrangement, however, have an increased risk for unbalanced gametes. Examples of balanced rearrangements include translocations and inversions.

Translocations

> Translocations involve the exchange of genetic material between nonhomologous chromosomes.

There are two types of translocations, reciprocal and Robertsonian.

Reciprocal translocations

> Reciprocal translocations involve the breakage of nonhomologous chromosomes with reciprocal exchange of chromosome material.

The carrier of a reciprocal translocation is usually phenotypically normal (unless a gene or genes have been disrupted by the translocation). However, carriers have an increased risk for unbalanced gametes and abnormal phenotype in their offspring.

An example is shown, in Figure 7-5, of the meiotic segregation patterns that are possible in the carrier of a balanced, reciprocal translocation. In this particular example, the parent carries a reciprocal translocation between the terminal short arms of chromosomes 1 and 3. The breakpoints are at chromosomes 1p31 and 3p21. Notice that the two translocation chromosomes form an unusual

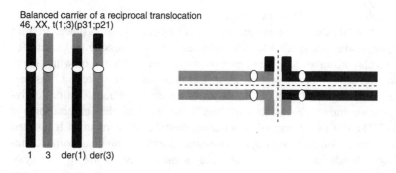

Balanced carrier of a reciprocal translocation
46, XX, t(1;3)(p31;p21)

1   3   der(1) der(3)

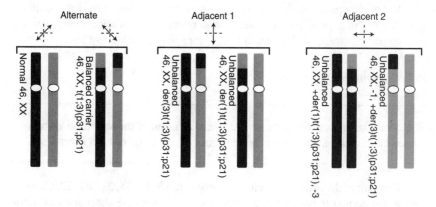

Alternate   Adjacent 1   Adjacent 2

Normal 46, XX

Balanced carrier
46, XX, t(1;3)(p31;p21)

Unbalanced
46, XX, der(3)t(1;3)(p31;p21)

Unbalanced
46, XX, der(1)t(1;3)(p31;p21)

Unbalanced
46, XX, +der(1)t(1;3)(p31;p21), −3

Unbalanced
46, XX, −1, +der(3)t(1;3)(p31;p21)

Figure 7-5 Synapse formation and segregation of a balanced reciprocal chromosome translocation.

"quadriradial" synapse with the normal homolog of chromosomes 1 and 3. The quadriradial synapse may be resolved in one of three ways. Alternate segregation yields one gamete with a normal complement of chromosomes and another gamete containing the pair of reciprocally balanced translocation chromosomes. Each of these gametes should produce an individual with a normal phenotype following fertilization by a normal gamete of the opposite sex. Either of the adjacent segregation patterns, however, yields unbalanced gametes. Each gamete contains a partial trisomy and a partial monosomy, and is expected on fertilization to produce an abnormal phenotype. The nomenclature used to describe the expected conception products is listed. Let's take the product on the far right of the figure, 46, XX, −1, +der(3)t(1;3)(p31;p21) as an example. The first position indicates the total number of chromosomes, which is 46. The next position indicates the sex chromosomes complement; we will arbitrarily suppose that this abnormal gamete is maternally derived and becomes fertilized by a normal sperm containing an X chromosome. Thus, the expected conception will be female with a normal complement of sex chromosomes (XX). A (+) or (−) sign is placed in front of a chromosome as a symbol to indicate an extra (+) or missing (−) normal or abnormal chromosome. Note that chromosomes are named based on which chromosome the centromere is derived from. Chromosome 1 is, therefore, missing, and we indicate this fact with "1." In its place, however, is a translocation "derivative" chromosome (abbreviated as "der"), so we call this chromosome a "der(3)." The last two pieces of information describe the derivative. It resulted from a translocation (t) involving chromosomes 1 and 3, with breakpoints corresponding to bands 1p31 and 3p21. There are some nuances in the logic of cytogenetic nomenclature, and the standards change from time-to-time; so, it is not worth getting too hung up on the details, however.

It would appear that the risk of producing an abnormal offspring would be quite high (2 in 3, or 67%); however, due to prenatal loss of abnormal offspring, the empiric recurrence risk is much lower (approximately 5% to 15%).

Robertsonian translocations

Robertsonian translocations are the result of fusion of the long arms of two acrocentric chromosomes at the centromeres, with loss of both short arms.

Remember the acrocentric chromosomes are 13, 14, 15, 21, and 22. Carriers of a Robertsonian translocation are usually normal because short arms of acrocentric chromosomes contain redundant copies of ribosomal RNA genes, and, thus, no essential genetic material is lost. However, carriers are at risk for producing conceptions with monosomy or trisomy. An example of meiotic segregation of a Robertsonian translocation is given in the Down syndrome section (Fig. 7-4). The empiric risk for abnormal phenotype in the offspring of a Robertsonian translocation carrier female is 10% to 15%; and in a male it is 1% to 2%.

The observed frequency of abnormal phenotypes resulting from unbalanced chromosome segregation in the children of a parent with a balanced reciprocal translocation or Robertsonian translocation is always less than the theoretical, predicted frequency. This, presumably, results from high rates of early fetal wastage for unbalanced conceptions. The risk of having unbalanced offspring is less for male carriers of a balanced translocation than it is for female carriers and presumably reflects ineffective spermatogenesis.

Recurrent miscarriage is one indication that either parent is a carrier of a balanced rearrangement, and the spontaneously aborted conceptions represent the products of unbalanced segregation.

Inversions

Inversions result from two breaks on a chromosome with inversion of the segment and reinsertion at its original site.

Inversions that involve the centromere are called "pericentric." Inversions that do not involve the centromere are termed "paracentric."

Approximately 1 in 1000 individuals carries an inversion. Inversions are balanced structural rearrangements and inversion carriers are usually phenotypically normal (no loss or gain of genetic material). However, carriers are at risk to produce offspring with deletions or duplications and resultant abnormal phenotype. During pairing of homologous chromosomes in meiosis, a chromosome with an inversion will form a loop to line up correctly with its homolog (Fig. 7-6). If crossing over occurs within the loop, resultant gametes may have duplications or deletions of chromosome material. Individuals with a pericentric

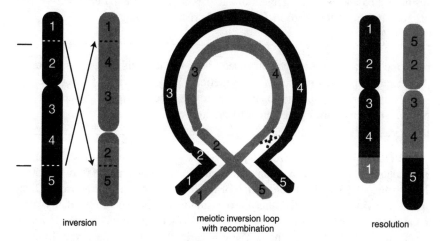

inversion   meiotic inversion loop   resolution
                            with recombination

Figure 7-6   Consequences of pericentric inversion.

inversion have a 5% to 15% risk of producing a child with an abnormal phenotype. This risk is much less ($< 1\%$) for those individuals carrying a paracentric inversion, because most abnormal chromosomes are dicentric or acentric and therefore lead to a nonviable conception. (The outstanding student may be able to draw the equivalent of Fig. 7-6 for a paracentric inversion.)

Deletions

> Deletions are caused by a break in a chromosome with resultant loss of chromosome material.

> Breaks leading to the loss of the chromosome tip are called terminal deletions. Interstitial deletions refer to a loss of genetic material between two breaks within a chromosome.

Deletions result in an abnormal phenotype, presumably due to the loss of one or more genes.

A well-documented terminal deletion syndrome is Cri-du-Chat syndrome (5p−). Infants with Cri-du-Chat syndrome have a very distinctive "cat-like" cry as well as microcephaly, growth retardation, and a unique facial appearance. These individuals have profound mental retardation. Most cases are de novo chromosome abnormalities; however, approximately 10% to 15% may be the result of a balanced rearrangement in one parent. Therefore, parental karyotypes are recommended for appropriate recurrence risk counseling.

> Some deletions are too small to see under the light microscope and are detectable only by molecular cytogenetic techniques such as fluorescence in situ hybridization (FISH). We refer to these conditions as "microdeletion" (or contiguous gene deletion) syndromes.

Velocardiofacial syndrome (VCFS) is probably the most common microdeletion syndrome, with an estimated incidence of 1 in 3000 to 1 in 5000 live births. VCFS is due to a deletion of the long arm of one chromosome 22 at q11.2. Individuals with VCFS may have a submucous or overt cleft palate (velo), conotruncal heart disease (cardio), distinctive facial features (facial), learning problems, and psychiatric illness. There is variability of the phenotype. In other words, some individuals with this microdeletion are mildly affected, whereas others are more severely affected. VCFS is inherited in an autosomal dominant fashion, and, therefore, affected individuals have a 50% chance of having a child with VCFS with each pregnancy. Interestingly, DiGeorge syndrome (DGS), a condition once thought to be separate and distinct from VCFS, is also caused by a deletion of the 22q11.2 region in the majority of patients. Individuals with DGS have conotruncal heart disease, hypoplastic/absent thymus with resultant immune deficiency, and hypoplastic/absent parathyroid glands with resultant hypocalcemia.

One reason for variability in microdeletion syndromes is that different individuals will each have a deletion of varying extents involving different flanking genes (Fig. 7-7). Nevertheless, a common collection of overlapping phenotypes, resulting from overlapping regions of deletion, can be identified.

Duplications

Chromosome duplications are simply a duplicated region of genetic material resulting in a partial trisomy.

Duplications result in an abnormal phenotype. Duplications of chromosome material may result from unequal crossing-over during meiosis or may occur in the offspring of reciprocal translocation carriers.

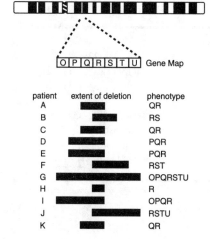

Figure 7-7 Interindividual variability in a microdeletion (also known as a contiguous gene deletion) syndrome.

CANCER CYTOGENETICS

Acquired chromosome abnormalities may occur in various types of hematologic malignancies and solid tumors. These are chromosome rearrangements in somatic cells that can alter the position of various genes and subsequently, alter the gene product. This alteration may then cause malignancy. An example of this type of phenomenon is the reciprocal translocation between chromosomes 9 and 22, seen in patients with chronic myelogenous leukemia (CML). This translocation alters the position of a proto-oncogene causing an altered gene product and resultant leukemia. The derivative chromosome 22 is referred to as the "Philadelphia chromosome," and is a marker for CML.

Some common leukemias and solid tumors and their associated chromosome aberrations are listed in Table 7-4. These very specific chromosome differences are helpful in the diagnosis, prognosis, and management of cancer patients. They may also help define periods of relapse and remission based on the presence or absence of the chromosome aberration.

TABLE 7-4
SELECTED CYTOGENETIC ABNORMALITIES
CHARACTERISTICALLY ASSOCIATED
WITH PARTICULAR NEOPLASMS

CONDITION	TYPICAL ABERRATION
Leukemias	
Acute myeloblastic	t(8;21)(q22;q22)
Acute promyelocytic(M3)	t(15;17)(q22;q11-12)
Chronic myelogenous	t(9;22)(q34;q11)
Solid tumors	
Burkitt's lymphoma	t(8;14)(q24;q32)
Meningioma	monosomy 22
Retinoblastoma	del(13)(q14)
Wilms' tumor	del(11)(p13)

INDICATIONS FOR A CHROMOSOME ANALYSIS

So, when is it appropriate to order a chromosome analysis? The following are examples of individuals who may have a chromosome abnormality or carry a rearrangement that may predispose to offspring with a chromosome abnormality.

- Individuals with multiple congenital malformations, mental retardation, and growth failure (typical characteristics of an autosomal chromosomal imbalance).
- Individuals with suspected chromosome abnormalities based on their phenotype (confirmatory testing).
- Couples with multiple pregnancy loss (suspecting that one parent may carry a balanced rearrangement).
- Females with short stature or primary amenorrhea (possible X chromosome abnormality, i.e., Turner's syndrome).
- Males with infertility (possibly Klinefelter's syndrome or Y chromosome abnormality).
- Patients with ambiguous genitalia (to confirm genotype).
- Patients with hematologic malignancies (to aid in diagnosis of a specific malignancy based on the type of acquired chromosome abnormality).

PRENATAL DIAGNOSIS TECHNIQUES

Prenatal diagnosis has three uses. First, it can be used as the basis for parental decision making in determining whether to continue or electively terminate the pregnancy. Second, it can detect fetal disease that, increasingly, is amenable to prenatal therapeutic medical and surgical intervention. Third, the diagnostic information can be used to educate the parents with respect to what birth defects are likely to be encountered and what sort of developmental issues will be faced in early childhood and beyond.

TRIPLE SCREEN

The triple screen is a maternal blood test used to screen for Down syndrome and also trisomy 18 and neural tube defects. The test is performed around the 16th week of pregnancy.

The triple screen assays the values of three "analytes," maternal serum alpha-fetoprotein (AFP), unconjugated estriol (uE3), and human chorionic gonadotropin (HCG). The test results are recorded as a multiple of the normal median (MoM) for a given gestational age. In Down syndrome, maternal serum AFP and uE3 are depressed but levels of HCG are elevated. It is only about 65% sensitive for all maternal ages, however, and it will have a significant false negative rate. Ultrasound does not add to the sensitivity of the screen for Down syndrome. If the test is positive, then amniocentesis and karyotype should be offered. In trisomy 18, all three analytes are low, and the sensitivity is about 75%. In neural tube defects (open spina bifida and anencephaly), maternal serum AFP will be elevated.

AMNIOCENTESIS

Amniocentesis is a method of obtaining fetal amniotic cells for karyotype. It is typically performed at 15 to 20 weeks' gestation.

Amniocentesis can always be performed later in gestation, but the fetal cells do not grow as well. It is invasive, and the risk for fetal loss is best quoted as 1 in 200. Amniotic AFP can also more sensitively detect neural tube defects. Complications include, in addition to fetal loss, chorioamnionitis and rupture of membranes. All procedures are done with ultrasound visualization, and 20 to 30 mL of amniotic fluid are typically aspirated from the amniotic cavity.

Amniocentesis with karyotype is recommended for all pregnant women at age 35 years and above.

The risk for Down syndrome greatly accelerates at maternal age $\geq$ 35 years. It should be kept in mind, however, that only about 20% of all children with Down syndrome are born to mothers of this age or older (because the majority of all children are born to younger mothers). As a screening measure, then, this approach fails to detect the majority of fetuses at risk for Down syndrome.

CHORIONIC VILLUS SAMPLING (CVS)

> CVS is essentially a placental biopsy and is performed at about 10 to 12 weeks' gestation.

CVS is no longer routinely performed before 10 weeks because of a risk for limb reduction defects. Two methods are used, transcervical and transabdominal. Compared to amniocentesis, it has a higher rate of fetal loss ($\sim1\%$), risk for late complications including secondary oligohydramnios ($\sim1\%$), failure to obtain fetal tissue ($\sim1\%$), tendency toward ambiguous cytogenetic results or maternal cell contamination ($\sim1\%$ to 2%), and a higher laboratory culture failure rate ($\sim2\%$).

PERCUTANEOUS UMBILICAL BLOOD SAMPLING (PUBS)

> PUBS is a method of directly sampling fetal blood and is performed after 18 weeks' gestation. It is the fastest method for obtaining a fetal karyotype.

Under ultrasound guidance, a needle is inserted into the umbilical vein of the umbilical cord. A major advantage of the technique is that a karyotype can be performed directly, and hence, rapidly from fetal leukocytes, in contrast to amniocentesis and CVS, in which it takes some time for the sample of fetal cells to be cultured. There is a 1% risk for miscarriage or fetal death, so this method should only be used if the diagnosis cannot be made by amniocentesis or CVS or if a rapid cytogenetic diagnosis is required. PUBS may also be used to diagnose fetal infections or hematological problems or as a means to transfuse blood components or inject medication.

COMPLEX INHERITANCE[†]

•

- The Threshold Model

  The Effects of Genes

  The Effect of Environment

  The Effect of Genes and Environment

  Sex Dependence of the Threshold

  Other Characteristics of Complex Inheritance

•   •   •   •   •   •   •   •   •   •   •   •

The vast majority of diseases do not result from single gene, mendelian inheritance. Nevertheless, from twin studies and other studies documenting familial aggregation, there clearly is a genetic contribution to the risk for many common diseases, including hypertension, atherosclerotic vascular disease, obesity, diabetes mellitus, mental illness, alcoholism, Alzheimer's disease, multiple sclerosis, many birth defects, and other illnesses.

> Instead of a single gene, most diseases result from a combination of genes, each contributing an additive risk, in combination with environmental exposures.

It should be pointed out, as well, that the majority of non-pathologic traits that distinguish people—personality; intelligence; habitus; skin, hair, and eye color; facial appearance; and so forth—are likely inherited in a similarly complex fashion. Several, at times confusing and somewhat overlapping, terms are used to describe these phenomena:

[†]The organization of this chapter benefitted from a lecture outline developed by Dr. Gail Jarvik at the University of Washington.

Polygenic inheritance: Generally, this implies that the disease is the result of the additive effects of multiples of different genes, each of which, acting alone, would be insufficient to cause the disease. Each of the contributory genes may not have an equal weight; some may have major effects in conferring risk for the disease, whereas others might weigh in with relatively minor contributions.

Complex inheritance: This term is used to convey the fact that the disease can result from a variety of different causes. It may be the result of a single gene inherited in a mendelian manner; it may be the result of the additive effects of several genes (i.e., polygenic); it may have environmental etiologies, such as diet, infectious agents, or trauma; or in any particular individual, it might result from a combination of some or all of the above. It is usually used interchangeably with the term "multifactorial inheritance."

EXAMPLE: ALZHEIMER'S DISEASE

Alzheimer's disease, like most common diseases, demonstrates complex inheritance. Having a first degree relative (parent, sibling, or child) increases one's risk for developing Alzheimer's disease by about two- to three-fold. There are rare families that inherit a predisposition to Alzheimer's disease as an autosomal dominant disorder resulting from mutation in one of three known genes (presinilin 1, presinilin 2, or beta amyloid precursor protein). In most families, no simple mendelian pattern of inheritance can be discerned, however, and the combination of genes at several loci contributes to the risk for the disease. One of those contributory genes is apoliprotein E. Three alleles are known, e1, e2, and e3. The e2 allele is protective. The e4 allele confers elevated risk. Homozygotes for the e2 allele have the lowest risk, whereas individuals homozgyous for the e4 allele have the highest risk. Nevertheless, the majority of e4 homozygous individuals still do not develop Alzheimer's disease, yet many people homozygous for the e2 allele still do. There is good evidence that other genes contribute to the risk for Alzheimer's disease, too. An individual's genotype at these other, still largely undetermined, loci accounts, in part, for the observation that the apoliprotein E genotype is contributory—but by no means solely determinative—of whether an individual will develop Alzheimer's disease or not. Finally, at least one environmental factor, head injury, is associated with a risk for Alzheimer's disease. In any given individual with Alzheimer's disease, it is likely that all or a subset of these factors caused the disease. Even in those rare people who inherit risk for Alzheimer's disease in an autosomal dominant manner, other genes, like apoliprotein E, and environmental exposures probably account for variable expressivity (as exemplified by a differing age of onset and tempo of progression between individuals, even those within the same family who inherit the same mutation).

THE THRESHOLD MODEL

Complex inheritance is fairly well explained by the threshold model.

THE EFFECT OF GENES

We begin by applying the threshold model to the subset of cases resulting from polygenic inheritance (in which we initially exclude an environmental contribution). We suppose that two loci contribute equally to the risk for developing a particular disease, say, age related hearing loss. One gene, which we call gene A, has two alleles of equal frequency, allele 0 and allele 1. Allele 0 confers no risk for hearing loss and allele 1 does confer risk for hearing loss. We further suppose that each of the alleles acts additively, in that genotype 0/0 has no risk, genotype 1/1 has the highest risk, and genotype 1/0 confers an intermediate level of risk. We will call the other locus, gene B, and also give it two equally frequent alleles, 0 and 1, with the same properties as gene A. The degree of risk conferred by allele 1 of gene A equals the same amount of risk as conferred by allele 1 of gene B. As shown in Figure 8-1, there are sixteen possible segregation patterns for each of the two alleles of the A and B genes. There are actually only eight distinct genotypes, but some of them can be redundantly generated. By merely adding the number of allele number 1s at each of the two loci, note that there are five categories of risk, ranging from zero risk (homozygous zero for each of A and B) to risk level 4 (homozygous 1 for each of A and B). There are four equally probable different combinations (resulting in two distinct genotypes) that achieve each of risk level 3 and risk level 1. There are six equally probable different combina-

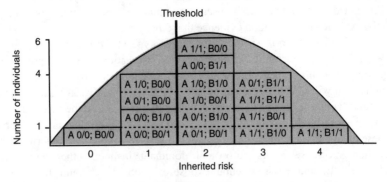

Figure 8-1   Threshold model for inherited risk.

tions (resulting in three different genotypes) to achieve risk level 2. Thus, we generate this distribution curve, with the most frequent category of genotype in the population being one with risk level 2 and the rarest genotypes being ones with zero risk or risk level 4.

Now, suppose that age related hearing loss happens when some "threshold" level of risk is crossed, here arbitrarily set as greater than or equal to risk level 2, such that 11 in 16 (69%) members of the population become partly deaf by a certain age. In our simple, hypothetical two gene model, it can be seen that some individuals will cross the threshold of risk merely as a consequence of their genotype at gene A (being homozygous for allele 1). For others, their genotype at gene B (homozygous for allele 1) will be sufficient to push them over the threshold. For others still, who have milder genotypes at each locus (heterozygous for allele 1 at both gene A and gene B), the sum of contributions from both gene A and gene B will push them past the threshold. For many complex diseases, remember that there are likely to be more than two contributory genes, with more than two alleles for each gene, and not each gene and each allele will possess equal weight.

We could also measure the phenotype a bit more quantitatively than saying that someone is either hard of hearing or is not hard of hearing. In fact, many phenotypes, such as body weight, height, blood pressure, cholesterol levels, and so forth, can be quantified, and more statistically sophisticated methods have been developed to evaluate them.

THE EFFECT OF ENVIRONMENT

To make the model a bit more complete, we throw environmental factors into the brew. Exposure to occupational noise is one non-genetic factor that influences risk for hearing loss. For simplicity, we will score the severity of exposure to noise on a scale of 0 to 5, with 5 being worst, and assume a bell-shaped distribution curve for noise exposure in the population. We get a curve (Fig. 8-2) that looks similar to the one for our two locus polygenic model. (In reality, this curve

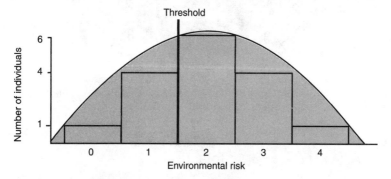

Figure 8-2   Threshold model for environmental risk.

can take on any shape, depending on how the environmental exposure is distributed in the population.) Thus, we could also envision some threshold exposure of noise that would lead to deafness, just as we did with the previous, simple two gene polygenic example. Of course, there are other environmental exposures that contribute to deafness risk, such as aminoglycoside antibiotics.

THE EFFECT OF GENES AND ENVIRONMENT

But, what we really want to do is combine the effects of genes and environment. So, we merely make a 3-D curve, as shown in Figure 8-3. On one axis (X or

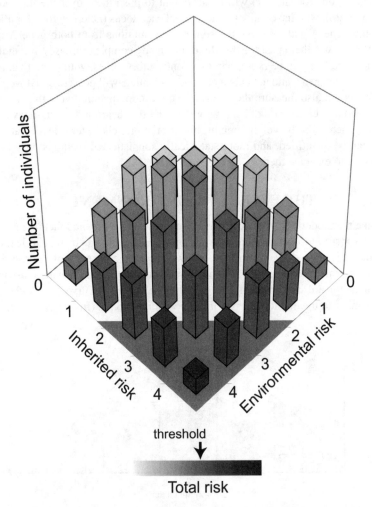

Figure 8-3   Threshold model considering both inherited and environmental risk.

length), we plot the environmental risk, and on the other axis (Y or depth), we plot the genetic risk. (On the Z or height axis, we have plotted the relative number of individuals in each particular category of gene and environmental risk.) The total risk is the sum of the genetic and environmental risk (here denoted by various shades of gray, with white representing the lowest risk of 0 and black representing the highest risk of 8). Now we can set the threshold at, say, a total level of 6. Anyone with a combined risk of 6 or greater will have the phenotype. It can be seen that nobody in our simple model becomes hard of hearing just from occupational exposure to noise alone, and nobody becomes hard of hearing just by what genes they inherit—again emphasizing that this is just a hypothetical example. Rather, it is the particular combination of genes and environment that accounts for the overall risk of age-related deafness. Individuals with a greater inherited risk will require less environmental exposure and, vice versa, individuals with more significant environmental exposure may develop the phenotype even with a relatively low risk genetic background.

> For a complex disease, a threshold level of environmental and genetic risk factors must be crossed to develop the disease. Not all genes contribute equally to risk in all people for a complex disease.

SEX DEPENDENCE OF THE THRESHOLD

In reality, the threshold for developing the disease may differ between men and women. For example, coronary artery disease is a complex disease resulting in rare circumstances from the influence of a single gene (such as the LDL receptor in familial hypercholesterolemia), but more often from a polygenic contribution (i.e., multiple genes influencing cholesterol and triglycerides) as well as environmental factors (such as diet, smoking, and exercise). For any given level of genetic and environmental risk, however, men have more coronary artery disease, because of the protective effects of estrogen in women. This means we should shift the threshold back and forth in our curves when we are discussing a particular sex.

> There is an interesting consequence of the fact that the risk threshold differs between the sexes: the recurrence risk in children will be greater for the children of the less susceptible sex.

For example, if your mother has coronary artery disease, you are at greater risk for developing coronary artery disease (regardless of your own sex), than if your father had coronary artery disease. Since women have a higher threshold for developing coronary artery disease, they must therefore have more risk factors overall and are, consequently, likely to have more genetic risk factors that you are capable of inheriting. You are, therefore, more likely to inherit more genetic risk factors from your mother than you would if it were your father who were affected.

OTHER CHARACTERISTICS OF COMPLEX INHERITANCE

> The recurrence risk for complex diseases is proportional to the population risk of the phenotype.

The more "disease genes" in the population, the more likely the recurrence risk in the offspring. This simply results from the fact that there is an increased probability of disease genes being brought in from more than one family member, such as both parents, instead of just one.

> The recurrence risk for complex diseases is lower for second-degree relatives (aunt, uncle, nephew, niece, grandparent, or grandchild) than for first-degree relatives, and continues to decline rapidly as the relationship becomes more distant.

Since multiple predisposing genes are needed to be affected, second-degree relatives are much less likely to get all these genes than first-degree relatives. For example, at a single locus, a child has a 1 in 2 probability of inheriting a high risk allele from one locus from a parent. The child would have a 1 in 4 probability for inheriting a second high risk allele from a second locus $\left(\frac{1}{2} \times \frac{1}{2} = \left(\frac{1}{2}\right)^2 = \frac{1}{4}\right)$. If there were n loci contributing to the risk for the disease, the risk for inheriting a high risk allele from all n loci would be $\left(\frac{1}{2}\right)^n$ for first-degree relative pairs. On the other hand, an individual's risk of inheriting a high risk allele from a grandparent is just 1 in 4; the probability for inheriting a second high risk allele from a second locus from the grandparent will be just 1 in 16 $\left(\frac{1}{4} \times \frac{1}{4} = \frac{1}{16}\right)$. If there were n loci contributing to the risk, then the risk for inheriting a high risk allele from all n loci would be $\left(\frac{1}{4}\right)^n$ for second-degree relative pairs. It can be seen in Figure 8-4 that the slope of the curve for second-degree relatives is much steeper than that for first-degree relatives. For third-degree relatives, such as first cousins, who share only $\frac{1}{8}$ of their genes in common, the risk drops off by the relationship $\left(\frac{1}{8}\right)^n$, which results in only minimal recurrence risk. It is also reasonable to expect first-degree

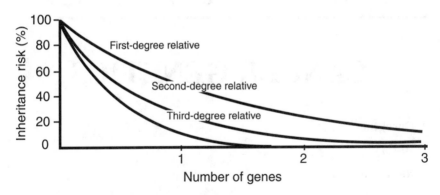

Figure 8-4   Weak recurrence risk among distant relatives for polygenic traits.

relatives to share more common environments than for more distantly related family members who do not live together.

> The recurrence risk for complex diseases is higher when more than one family member is affected.

It makes sense that the more people affected in a family, the more predisposing genes there will be in the family, and, consequently, the greater the risk of transmission from either or both parent(s).

Fortunately, we rarely have to resort to these theoretical considerations. Usually, we can just find a table from a prior epidemiologic study to look up empiric recurrence risk based on the number of affected parents and/or siblings. Illustrated in Table 8-1, is the risk for the recurrence of cleft lip, with or without cleft palate, a birth defect that is inherited in a complex fashion.

TABLE 8-1
RECURRENCE RISK FOR CLEFT LIP +/− CLEFT PALATE (%)

NUMBER SIBS AFFECTED	NEITHER PARENT AFFECTED	ONE PARENT AFFECTED	BOTH PARENTS AFFECTED
0	0.1	3	34
1	3	11	40
2	8	19	45

· C H A P T E R · 9 ·

CANCER GENETICS
·

There are three types of cancer genes: oncogenes, tumor suppressor genes, and DNA repair/cell cycle genes.

There is some overlap within each category; however, each of the three groups followed relatively different historical paths to discovery, and each has a somewhat unique clinical function.

ONCOGENES

HISTORY

The first hint of the existence of oncogenes was the observation in 1911 by Peyton Rous that a virus can cause sarcoma in chickens. In 1970 Howard Temin and David Baltimore independently discovered that the genome of the Rous sarcoma virus—and other "retroviruses" like it—is composed of RNA and that a unique enzyme, reverse transcriptase, reverse transcribes the RNA into DNA on infection in the cells of its host animal.

The reverse transcription of RNA to DNA in retroviruses represents a noteworthy violation of the "central dogma" of molecular biology.

Subsequently, it was demonstrated that retroviruses were capable of cellular "transformation" when infected in vitro into cells growing in tissue culture. Transformation refers to the process of an individual cell behaving like a tumor cell, in which the transformed cell displays aggressive growth characteristics, such as failing to inhibit its growth on contact with neighboring cells—the usual property of a well behaved, non-transformed, non-tumor cell growing in culture. In 1976, Michael Bishop and Harold Varmus discovered that the gene in a retrovirus that is responsible for cellular transformation is a mutant version of a gene found in the host organism. Working with the Rous sarcoma virus, they identified a gene src from the chicken that also has a closely conserved homolog in all animals. The non-mutated form of the gene, as it is found in the host organism, is known as a "proto-oncogene".

Another milestone in oncogene research was the discovery in 1979 by Robert Weinberg that in many human tumors—in which there is no evidence of retroviral infection—the very same oncogenes of retroviruses are also mutated and that they are once again capable of leading to cellular transformation. How the experiments were performed is illustrated in Figure 9-1. DNA was extracted from a human tumor. The DNA was then used to "transfect" non-malignant mouse cells growing in culture. (Transfection is the process of getting a cell to take up foreign DNA under experimental culture conditions. Often, the DNA can randomly integrate into the genome of the host cell.) It was then observed that a few rare clones of the transfected mouse cells were transformed (that is, grew in vitro with tumor-like properties), presumably because they happened to be transfected with a particular mutant gene from the tumor that is capable of causing cellular transformation. It is possible to separate human from mouse DNA using hybridization methods like Southern blots because the transfected fragment will include repetitive sequences that are unique to each species. When this was done, it was found that cellular transformation in mouse cells resulted from transfection of a mutated version of a human proto-oncogene, whose evolutionarily related homolog in other species was known from earlier studies as the transforming gene of a retrovirus capable of inducing cancer in some animal models. This experiment was significant for proving that the same oncogenes responsible for retrovirus-induced transformation were similarly mutated in human tumors resulting from nonviral causes.

RETROVIRUS STRUCTURE

The molecular anatomy of retroviruses is now well understood (Fig. 9-2). They have three genes: gag, pol, and env. Gag and env encode proteins that form the core and envelope, respectively, of the viral particle, while pol encodes the reverse transcriptase. The three genes are flanked by repetitive sequences (long terminal repeats, known as the LTR) that contain a promoter responsible for initiating transcription. The lifestyle of the retrovirus is as follows.

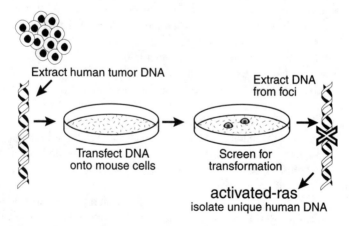

Figure 9-1   Weinberg transformation assay.

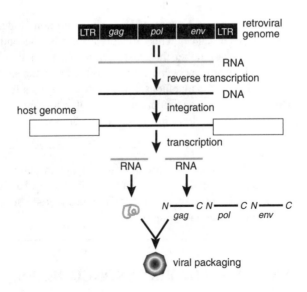

Figure 9-2 Retrovirus life cycle.

1. The virions enter cells.
2. The RNA genome is reverse transcribed by the viral reverse transcriptase into a DNA copy.
3. The DNA copy randomly integrates somewhere in the host cell's DNA. (This is called a provirus and the virus's genome is now known as a pro-genome.)
4. The viral infection can persist in this stage indefinitely, all the while using the cellular RNA polymerase to run off RNA copies of its genome, some of which are translated into more viral particles and some of which get packaged into that viral particle.

    The mature retroviral particles are then free to infect other cells and complete their life cycle all over again in a new host. On rare occasions, the virus manages to infect a cell in the germline and the provirus is transmitted to one's offspring, with mendelian segregation, just like any other gene.

    At some low frequency, however, the RNA retroviral genome can become fused with a cellular gene. This presumably happens when a normal cellular mRNA somehow gets mistakenly packaged with the viral RNA and the two molecules later recombine. No matter how this happens, this process of a retrovirus grabbing a cellular gene and packaging it is called transduction.

    As it turns out, retroviruses can be a major cause of cancer in animals (such as feline leukemia virus), but are an extremely rare cause of cancer in humans. [Human T cell leukemia virus I (HTLV1) causes a unique form of leukemia in Japan and is probably the only example of this. Human immunodeficiency virus

(HIV), which is a retrovirus, is a cause of Hodgkin's and non-Hodgkin's lymphoma, both being forms of cancer. This probably results as a secondary consequence of immunodeficiency rather than direct viral transformation, per se, as HIV does not ever pick up any oncogenes.] On the other hand, the study of retroviruses remains valuable, as the mutations in the proto-oncogenes first identified in non-human retroviruses are an important contributor to cancer in humans. Most human tumors do, in fact, have mutations in one or more proto-oncogenes.

> Retroviruses are not a significant cause of cancer in humans, although they are in other animals. The main medical value of their study has been the identification of cellular proto-oncogene homologues that are somatically mutated in many non-hereditary tumors.

EXAMPLES OF PROTO-ONCOGENES

Many mammalian proto-oncogenes are known (Table 9-1). Oncogenes can usually be fitted within a cellular pathway in which they have a role regulating growth and differentiation.

In contrast to tumor suppressor genes (as we will soon discuss), the mutations that turn a proto-oncogene into a cancer causing oncogene act dominantly at the cellular level. That is, one mutant copy of the oncogene is sufficient to participate in cellular transformation, and the normal, non-mutated version of the oncogene is insufficient to halt the process. Several different types of mutations

TABLE 9-1
ONCOGENES IDENTIFIED FROM ANIMAL RETROVIRUSES

ONCOGENE	VIRUS	PROTEIN
src	Chicken sarcoma virus	Tyrosine protein kinase
erbB	Avian erythroblastosis virus	EFG receptor/tyrosine protein kinase
erbA	Avian erythroblastosis virus	Throid homone receptor
ras	Murine sarcoma virus	GTPase
sis	Feline sarcoma virus	PDGF
fos	Murine osteosarcoma virus	jun with fos forms AP1 transcription factor
jun	Avian sarcoma virus	
myc	Avian myelocytomatosis virus	Transcription factor

can turn a proto-oncogene into an oncogene (Fig. 9-3). These include point mutation, translocations that lead to gene fusion events, translocations that lead to over
expression by placing the proto-oncogene under the inappropriate transcriptional
control of another gene's promoter or enhancer sequences, and gene amplification (in which a gene is duplicated in tandem several times, thereby increasing its
expression). The chromosome 9;22 translocation, which produces the Philadelphia chromosome in CML, results in a fusion of the protein coding sequences of
the bcr and abl proto-oncogones. Note that all of these processes lead either to an
altered gene product (with "gain of function" properties) or enhanced expression
of the gene. Deletion, or "loss of function," type mutations are not observed with
oncogenes.

Unlike tumor suppressor genes, mutations in proto-oncogenes are always
somatic and never inherited. (Although there are two exceptions, RET and
MET.)

It is important to emphasize that proto-oncogenes are activated by somatic
mutation. There are, of course, exceptions to every rule; there are two inherited
cancer predisposition syndromes that do result from germline transmission of a
mutant proto-oncogene. One is multiple endocrine neoplasia 2 (MEN2), in which
inherited mutations of the RET proto-oncogene can cause a syndrome in which
there is a high frequency of medullary thyroid carcinoma, parathyroid adenoma,
and pheochromocytoma of the adrenal and related tissue. The other is familial
renal cell carcinoma resulting from autosomal dominant inheritance of the MET
proto-oncogene. True to form, RET or MET can behave as traditional proto-

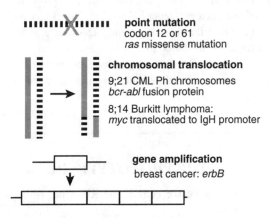

Figure 9-3 Activation of proto-oncogenes by mutation.

oncogenes and are often somatically mutated in individuals who have the non-inherited, correspondingly sporadic forms of these malignancies.

One final point. Oncogenes of retroviruses are distinct from the oncogenes of DNA tumor viruses. The oncogenes of DNA tumor viruses, unlike those of retroviruses, are unique to the virus and do not have cellular homologs. A well-known DNA tumor virus is the papilloma virus, which is a cause of human cervical carcinoma.

SUMMARY OF ONCOGENES

- Identified as transforming genes of retroviruses.
- An activated form of a cellular gene (proto-oncogene).
- Dominant at cellular level, means only one allele need be mutated.
- Mutations are somatic and never inherited (except for RET and MET).
- Retroviruses cause cancer in animals, but are not a significant cause of cancer in humans.

TUMOR SUPPRESSOR GENES

Most tumor suppressor genes were identified from medical genetic studies conducted on rare families with an autosomal dominant inherited predisposition to tumors. It should be said that the majority of cancer does not result from mendelian, single-gene inheritance; it results from cumulative somatic mutations in proto-oncogenes, tumor suppressor genes, and DNA repair/cell cycle control genes, although there is probably also complex inheritance of risk factors. Nevertheless, for almost any particular type of cancer, there are rare families that clearly transmit a genetic risk for that cancer, which can be attributed to a single gene transmitted in a mendelian fashion. It was postulated, and now shown in numerous examples, that such families inherit a germline mutation in a gene that otherwise must undergo somatic mutation to promote tumor development in the far more common, sporadic (non-inherited) cases of the particular tumor.

THE PROTOTYPE: RB

The prototype tumor suppressor gene is the RB gene, isolated as the cause of familial retinoblastoma.

Knudson's "two-hit" model of tumorigenesis

In 1971, Alfred Knudson proposed the elegant "two hit" model of tumorigenesis to explain the epidemiology of retinoblastoma. Retinoblastoma is a tumor of the retinal epithelium usually presenting in childhood. Knudson observed that about 40% of patients with retinoblastoma had an onset in infancy or early childhood. Those cases also tended to be bilateral; more frequently had a positive family history in an affected parent; and were often associated with additional malignancy like osteosarcoma, melanoma, or other tumors later in life. The remaining 60% of cases had a much later age of onset, tended to be unilateral, almost never had a family history of the tumor, and were not associated with risk for additional types of tumors. Knudson correctly hypothesized that the 40% of cases with early onset, bilaterality, and risk for secondary types of tumors represented a germline mutation in a particular gene. The 60% of cases with later onset, unilaterality, and no risk of secondary tumors resulted from somatic mutation of the same gene. He coined the term "tumor suppressor gene" for this hypothesized gene.

Knudson's reasoning went something like this: Let us define a tumor suppressor gene as one that unlike an oncogene, which must be activated by mutation, must be *in*activated to cause cancer. (Since there are two copies of all autosomal genes, we require that both copies of a tumor suppressor gene must be inactivated in order to promote tumor development.) Suppose that the chance of an inactivating mutation in any particular gene (in our case the tumor suppressor gene) in any particular cell is one in a million (10^{-6}). What is the probability then of mutating both alleles of the same gene in any particular cell? It is just $10^{-6} \times 10^{-6}$, which equals 10^{-12}. That is a very small number, and it is not too likely that this will happen. In fact, even if there were a million cells, say in the retina, the probability of any cell sustaining two mutagenic events—hits—is only about one in a million. But, what happens if someone inherits a mutation that inactivates one copy of that gene, such that all of the cells of the body, including the retina and other tissues, have, from the moment of conception, already sustained the first hit? Then, the probability of the second hit is still one in a million. And, since there are about a million cells in the retinal epithelium, the chance that the second hit will occur is pretty good. That is what happens with autosomal dominant inheritance of an inactivating mutation in a single copy of the RB gene. Somatic mutation of both alleles of RB is a much rarer event. We predicted the chances of that happening to be about one in a million, and that is about how often retinoblastoma occurs in the general population.

The rest of the differences between sporadic and inherited forms of RB is pretty well explainable. The occurrence of multiple tumors in individuals inheriting constitutional mutations in RB is due to the fact that the second hit occurs with high probability. In fact, the second hit is a random event. Some unfortunate patients will develop two or three or more retinoblastomas, and a few lucky individuals will be non-penetrant and escape ever developing a tumor. The occurrence of other types of tumors in individuals inheriting constitutional mutations in RB results from the fact that all of the cells in the body harbor the mutation. Since loss of RB function can lead to the development of tumors in other tissues, individuals with inherited mutations in RB are at high risk for these secondary tumors (osteosarcomas, fibrosarcomas, and melanoma). Finally, since tumor development requires two somatic mutation events in individuals not inheriting a mutant RB gene, it makes sense that the longer one lives, the greater the probability of exposure to mutation; this explains the later age of onset of tumor development in non-inherited forms of RB.

Since the time of Knudson's work, the RB gene has been cloned and molecularly characterized. RB is a phosphoprotein that regulates transit through the cell cycle by complexing with transcription factors. Somatic mutations of RB occur in many different types of tumors, and it turns out to be one of the most important genes in regulating choices between orderly growth and differentiation of tissues.

It should be emphasized that some individuals without a family history of RB can still have a constitutional mutation in one allele of RB. By now you should be able to come up with an explanation for this on your own. (The answer is that these individuals represent new mutations.) Such a person is subject to all the risks that befall an individual with a hereditary form of RB, including the probability of 1 in 2 of transmitting it to each of their children.

Note that, in contrast to oncogenes, RB and other tumor suppressor genes act recessively at the cellular level. This means that the normal function of a tumor suppressor gene is to . . . well, you guessed it, suppress tumor formation. Only when function is completely lost, through mutations that inactivate both alleles, can tumor growth be promoted.

Remember that proto-oncogenes must gain an activity to become a full-fledged oncogene. Tumor suppressor genes must lose their activity to cause cancer.

Most of the mutations of tumor suppressor genes (either inherited or somatic) are deletions or point mutations that cripple their function. Deletions of tumor suppressor genes are probably most common. Consequently, there is a unique experimental signature of a mutagenic event in the genome that takes out a tumor suppressor gene. The name for this is loss of heterozygosity.

Loss of heterozygosity

Suppose that you have DNA from someone with a sporadic (that is, not inherited) RB tumor. We can obtain both tumor DNA and DNA from white blood cells in the peripheral blood. The tumor DNA should have a mutation in RB. The peripheral white blood cell DNA should not. The mutation in RB in the tumor is likely to be a deletion. So if you do a Southern blot or PCR with a polymorphic marker (able to distinguish both alleles of RB) very close to RB, and both copies of RB are deleted in the tumor, then the peripheral blood should show the two different parental alleles and the tumor should show nothing. Very often, however, you see a pattern (Fig. 9-4) in which one of the parental copies appears deleted in the tumor, whereas both are present in the constitutional genome (the DNA obtained from the blood). The name for this phenomenon is loss of heterozygosity (LOH). How can it be explained? Often, the mutation affecting the second allele is a smaller deletion that does not encompass the marker or is an inactivating point mutation, leading to the appearance of only one marker. Other times, the first mutation is a small deletion or point mutation that switches the gene off, but the second "hit" to the other allele of RB is a "gene conversion event." A gene conversion event is a mitotic recombination that replaces the non-mutated allele with the mutated allele. (In simple terms, some DNA repair mechanism goes awry, correctly detects a difference between the two copies of the RB allele in the cell, and decides to fix it, but chooses the mutant allele by mistake as the one to use as the template for correcting the error.) The result is that both alleles of the RB gene are now the same and are both mutant.

LOH also happens in inherited forms of RB. Let us say that the germline mutation resides on one of the parental alleles, and the second hit in the tumor (which is always somatic) is a deletion or gene conversion event (replacing the normal parent's allele with the mutant parent's allele). Then the result is that only one parental allele will be detectable in the tumor (and that allele will be from the one involving the affected parent, if there is one).

Constitutional Tumor

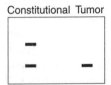

Figure 9-4   Loss of heterozygosity.

LOH is mostly useful from the research perspective. When LOH is present in a tumor from an individual in a family with an autosomal dominant inherited cancer predisposition syndrome, it confirms that the gene behaves as a tumor suppressor gene. When LOH is present in a tumor from an individual with a non-familial, sporadic malignancy, it suggests the presence of a tumor suppressor gene that has been somatically mutated.

RB microdeletion syndrome

Sometimes the deletions taking out RB on chromosome 13q14.1-q14.2 are quite large and involve other genes. There is thus a characteristic RB microdeletion syndrome that is seen in some individuals and has characteristic associated congenital abnormalities along with mental retardation. Some other tumor suppressor genes are also associated with microdeletion syndromes. Among these is the Wilms' tumor gene, WT1 on chromosome 11p13, responsible for the acronymic WAGR syndrome (Wilms' tumor, aniridia, genitourinary abnormalities, mental and growth retardation).

There are many inherited tumor suppressor gene syndromes. A nearly constant feature is that for every rare inherited syndrome, it turns out that in the sporadic, noninherited forms of the same type of tumor, the same tumor suppressor gene is mutated somatically. A constant feature of inherited tumor suppressor gene syndromes is that they are autosomal dominant.

P53 AND LI-FRAUMENI SYNDROME

p53 is a DNA-binding protein whose expression is induced by DNA damage. Among other things, it regulates decisions regarding "programmed" cell death (known as apoptosis). One molecular mechanism to reduce the probability of developing a tumor is to kill off cells that have sustained extensive mutation. Known as the "guardian of the genome," p53 monitors numerous signals recording the health of the cell. If it appears that enough mutations have accumulated to make it likely that the cell has undergone malignant transformation, p53 will make the decision to commit programmed cell death. But, what happens if p53 is not working? One can imagine that cells destined to form tumors will not be eliminated.

Germline mutations of p53 are the cause of the Li-Fraumeni syndrome. Li-Fraumeni syndrome is an autosomal dominant disorder involving the inheritance of multiple malignancies, especially breast cancer, soft tissue sarcomas, osteosarcoma, brain tumors, leukemia, and adrenocortical carcinoma.

Like RB, p53 is somatically mutated in many malignancies, especially colon cancer and small cell lung cancer, which, surprisingly, are not features of Li-Fraumeni syndrome.

NEUROFIBROMATOSIS 1

Neurofibromatosis 1 (NF1) is a common autosomal dominant inherited syndrome of benign tumors known as neurofibromas and other benign tumors of the peripheral and central nervous system. The tumors can occasionally undergo malignant transformation, and the spectrum of malignancy includes neurofibrosarcoma, schwannoma, glioma, pheochromocytoma, and leukemia. There are obvious cutaneous stigmata of the disease: the characteristic fleshy neurofibromas, hyperpigmented "cafe-au-lait" macules on the skin, raised hamartomatous lesions of the iris (Lisch nodules), and axillary and inguinal freckling. NF1 is caused by mutations in the neurofibromin gene, a GTPase-activating protein. Loss of its activity results in failure of hydrolysis of GTP to GDP. GTP is a common second messenger in intracellular signaling pathways. John Merrick, the "Elephant Man" popularized in a movie and whose remains were later purchased by the pop singer Michael Jackson, is commonly mistakenly said to have NF1. He almost certainly did not have NF1, but is thought to have had the proteus syndrome, a different disease entirely.

VON HIPPEL-LINDAU SYNDROME

The von Hippel-Lindau (VHL) syndrome is an autosomal dominant syndrome of benign vascular tumors of the cerebellum and retina (hemangioblastoma), pheochromocytoma, and renal cell cancer. As is the rule with most inherited tumor suppressor gene syndromes, both alleles of the gene responsible for familial VHL are nearly invariantly mutated in sporadic, non-familial forms of renal cell carcinoma (thus, demonstrating LOH). Interestingly, study of the rare cases of sporadic renal cell carcinoma not demonstrating LOH has allowed for the identification of yet another mechanism for inactivating a tumor suppressor gene. It turns out that in some individuals with renal cell carcinoma, a GC-rich region in the promoter becomes hypermethylated at the cytosines, switching off transcription of the gene and, thereby, leading to loss of expression without mutation.

FAMILIAL ADENOMATOUS POLYPOSIS

Familial adenomatous polyposis (FAP) is relatively common and accounts for about 1% of all cases of colon cancer. Individuals with FAP usually have their colons carpeted with polyps by no later than their teenage or early adult years.

Adenocarcinoma of the colon is inevitable, and prophylactic colectomy is the only treatment option. There are some "attenuated" forms of FAP that have a more limited extent of polyposis. There are occasionally extracolonic manifestations of the disease, including a characteristic fundoscopic lesion, CHRPE (congenital hypertrophy of the retinal pigment epithelium), and benign subcutaneous and bone cysts (known as the "Gardner syndrome," when present). The gene causing FAP is known as APC (for adenomatous polyposis coli), a protein with a complex role in cell cycle progression and extracellular communication and matrix attachment. To some degree, phenotype–genotype correlation is possible. That is, families with attenuated forms of FAP tend to have mutations that cluster within a confined region of the APC gene. As is the established paradigm with tumor suppressor genes, APC is commonly mutated in sporadic non-inherited forms of colon cancer. In fact, it's mutated in about half of all sporadic colon cancer. (As we'll soon discuss, the other half involve mutations in DNA mismatch repair genes, which were originally also defined by studies of rare families with colon cancer.)

Colon cancer, and in particular FAP, has proven to be one of the best tumors to study events responsible for malignancy. Complete progression from a single mutant cell to a full blown tumor requires the accumulation of numerous somatic mutations (regardless of whether the initial insult is inherited or sporadic). And other genes, including the ras proto-oncogene and p53, have significant roles. Thus, colon cancer, like other malignancies, evolves along a multi-step pathway in which cells become progressively malignant with the accumulation of new mutations.

FAMILIAL BREAST OR OVARIAN CANCER

Familial breast and ovarian cancer syndromes account for about 5% of all breast cancer. Familial breast cancer is genetically heterogeneous. Two genes are known, BRCA1 and BRCA2. There is undoubtedly at least a third locus that awaits discovery, as not all families with autosomal breast cancer have linkage to the BRCA1 or BRCA2 loci on chromosomes 17 and 13, respectively.

Breast cancer is a common disease, and about 1 in 9 of all North American women will develop it at some point in their lives. Thus, it is often hard to determine whether an individual case of breast cancer resulted from a familial predisposition or as a sporadic occurrence related to other causes (such as somatic mutation, environment, and polygenic inheritance).

Familial forms of breast cancer have several hallmarks, which help differentiate it from coincidental family clustering of sporadic cases. First, there tends to be a younger age of onset (often premenopausal). Second, bilateral occurrence of a tumor or multifocal occurrence of more than one primary on a single side (just as with inherited forms of retinoblastoma), tends to be somewhat more common in familial breast cancer. Third, the presence of ovarian cancer in a family, which is much rarer than breast cancer, is often suggestive of families inheriting BRCA1 mutations. Fourth, the occurrence of male breast cancer, a rare event, is associated with BRCA2 mutation. Conversely, even individuals from breast cancer families who turn out not to have inherited the predisposing gene can still get breast cancer as a sporadic disease (phenocopies).

Women inheriting a mutation in BRCA1 or BRCA2 face a lifetime risk of breast cancer of about 50% to 80%. Men do not usually get breast cancer when they inherit a BRCA1 mutation. However, men inheriting BRCA2 mutations are at elevated risk for developing breast cancer (approximately 6% lifetime risk). Women inheriting a BRCA1 mutation have a lifetime risk of ovarian cancer of approximately 25%, whereas the risk is much lower with BRCA2 mutations.

Germline, inherited BRCA1 mutation is associated with a greatly elevated risk for ovarian cancer. Because ovarian cancer, unlike breast cancer, is so uncommon in the general population, the specific elevated risk for ovarian cancer in BRCA1 is great. There is poor genotype–phenotype correlation with respect to developing ovarian cancer. That is, even if all the individuals in a family have developed exclusively breast cancer, it is still possible that the next affected woman could develop ovarian cancer (or vice versa). Germline mutations in both BRCA1 and BRCA2 may confer smaller elevations in risk for other types of tumors, but the genetic epidemiology is still a subject of investigation.

Some populations show founder effects for BRCA mutations.

About 2% of all Ashkenazi Jews are heterozygous for one of three different mutant alleles of either BRCA1 (two different alleles) or BRCA2 (one allele). Most familial breast and ovarian cancer in this population can be attributed to one of these three mutations.

Genetic testing for familial BRCA1 and BRCA2 mutations is revolutionizing the approach to this disease. Women found to inherit a germline mutation in either gene can consider treatment with the new anti-estrogen therapies (like tamoxifen) or consider undergoing prophylactic mastectomy and/or oophorectomy.

Typically, when an individual is tested for BRCA1 and BRCA2 mutations, the coding sequence of both genes are sequenced. For Ashkenazi Jewish individuals, it may be appropriate to begin with less expensive testing specifically evaluating for the presence of the three ancestral mutations, since these account for the majority of mutations observed in this population. Genetic testing turns out to be not quite so straightforward for BRCA1 and BRCA2. This is because both genes are large, the disease is allelically heterogeneous, and polymorphisms are frequent. Unless you have multiple affected members of the family available, it is not always so easy to determine if a subtle DNA sequence change (like a single basepair substitution causing a single amino acid substitution) represents a polymorphism of no particular significance or is the mutation causative of breast cancer in the family. On the other hand, as more and more individuals undergo genetic testing for BRCA1 and BRCA2 mutations, a large database of mutations and polymorphisms is being accumulated from different families, and this will help allow for determining the pathogenic significance of any particular observed sequence change.

Because of the complexities, both molecular and psychological, of BRCA mutation testing, genetic counseling is recommended before an individual is tested.

SUMMARY OF TUMOR SUPPRESSOR GENES

- Identified as genes responsible for autosomal dominant human tumor syndromes.
- Recessive at cellular level, means both alleles must be inactivated.
- Sporadic cases of the germ-line tumor often also show mutation, especially deletion or gene conversion events producing LOH.

DNA REPAIR/CELL CYCLE GENES

We know that somatic mutations of proto-oncogenes and somatic or inherited mutations of tumor suppressor genes lead to cancer, but what would happen if, rather than starting with a mutation in one of those genes, you began with a mutation in a gene responsible for maintaining the integrity of the genome? One might expect that somatic mutation of DNA repair and cell cycle control genes could lead to a cascade of mutations, eventually hitting proto-oncogenes and tumors suppressor genes responsible for cellular transformation—and that is precisely what happens. There are basically two types of genes in the category. One set of genes is directly involved in repairing DNA. The DNA molecule frequently undergoes physical damage. Bases are lost from the phosphodiester backbone. Bases become chemically modified by exposure to carcinogens and reactive oxygen species. There can be DNA strand breaks. Finally, DNA polymerase can mistakenly insert the wrong base, leading to a mismatch. Much of this damage can be directly fixed, and that job falls to the first category of genes. The second major category of gene is involved in recognizing that DNA damage or chromosomal abnormalities have occurred in the somatic cell, temporarily halting the cell division cycle until the damage can be fixed, and then making an assessment as to whether the cell was fixed properly and should either re-enter the cell cycle or commit programmed cell death. This latter "checkpoint" concept was introduced by Leland Hartwell in his seminal studies of yeast cell division mutants that failed to recognize when DNA damage had occurred. A checkpoint is a temporary stop in the cell cycle, at which a particular list of safeguards is monitored before going any further.

Several genes involved in DNA repair and regulation of the mitotic cell cycle have now been implicated as having a role in initiating cancer. Many of these genes are mutated in hereditary cancer predisposition syndromes.

AUTOSOMAL RECESSIVE SYNDROMES OF DEFICIENCY OF DNA REPAIR

The first group of DNA repair genes discovered to be involved in hereditary cancer predisposition syndromes is comprised of rare autosomal recessive syndromes of malignancy. They are each characterized by a cellular deficiency in various aspects of DNA repair. As a group, the study of these genes has suggested some important links between transcription and DNA repair, among other things.

1. **Bloom syndrome.** Mutations in a DNA helicase result in an increased frequency of mitotic sister chromatid exchanges (similar to meiotic recombination, except occurring during somatic cell division). Bloom syndrome individuals are at greatly elevated risk for hematopoietic malignancy.

2. **Xeroderma pigmentosum.** This is a genetically heterogeneous disorder, resulting from mutations in various transcription factors and nucleases. Individuals with xeroderma pigmentosum are at extreme risk for developing skin cancer on exposure to sunlight. This is due to a cellular defect in "excision repair" of ultraviolet light-induced thymidine dimers.

3. **Ataxia telangiectasia.** The defective gene in this disorder ordinarily recognizes broken chromosomes and participates in a cell cycle checkpoint to allow time for DNA repair. Affected individuals have a greatly elevated risk for hematopoietic and other malignancies. They also have a neurodegenerative syndrome characterized by an ataxic movement disorder, as well as cutaneous telangiectasias ("spider" malformations of small blood vessels).
4. **Fanconi anemia.** This is a genetically heterogeneous disease; several genes have been identified, so far with unknown function. Individuals with Fanconi anemia typically have a variety of birth defects, such as horseshoe kidney, and an extremely elevated risk for developing acute myelogenous leukemia.

HEREDITARY NONPOLYPOSIS COLORECTAL CANCER

Hereditary nonpolyposis colorectal cancer (HNPCC) involves susceptibility to numerous types of malignancy, most commonly of the colon and elsewhere in the GI tract, the endometrium, and the ovary. It is a genetically heterogeneous disease inherited in an autosomal dominant fashion. At least four different genes have now been identified, all involved in DNA double strand mismatch repair. The mismatches are incorrectly made basepairs that result from misinsertion of the wrong base by DNA polymerase during cellular replication. The two most common genes responsible for HNPCC are MSH2 and MLH1, with each being mutated in about a third of families with HNPCC. Mutations in the other genes are found only in rare families, and the culprit gene for nearly another third of HNPCC families still remains unknown. The DNA mismatch repair genes are extremely highly conserved between bacteria and higher mammals, suggesting an important role in basic cellular metabolism.

> Genomic instability of repeated sequences, known as microsatellite instability, is a hallmark of tumors from patients in HNPCC families.

This finding was first made when genetic linkage studies using polymorphic microsatellite markers were undertaken in HNPCC families. The surprising observation was that, instead of yielding a single band corresponding to one of the alleles for the marker, there was evident stuttering of the band on the gel, resulting from extremely frequent somatic mutation of the repetitive microsatellite sequences used as polymorphic markers in genetic linkage analysis (Fig. 9-5). The phenomenon is now understood to result directly from defective mismatch repair. Microsatellite instability is observed commonly in cancer, and

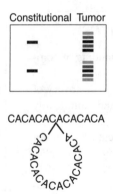

Figure 9-5   Microsatellite instability.

not just from tumors in individuals from HNPCC families; it is also seen in tumors from individuals without a hereditary predisposition to cancer.

The presence of microsatellite instability in a tumor indicates that the mismatch repair pathway in the cell has become defective.

In individuals without HNPCC, the mismatch repair gene is initially disabled by a somatic mutation, but once inactivated, it is capable of catalyzing further somatic mutation so that other genes become rapidly involved in an exploding cascade of mutation.

HNPCC accounts for about 5 to 10% of all cases of colon cancer. However, nearly half of colon cancers have evidence of microsatellite instability and somatic mutation of at least one mismatch repair gene. We previously noted that about half of all non-familial colon cancer had somatic mutation of the APC gene involved in FAP. Thus, nearly 100% of all non-inherited, sporadic cases of colon cancer are explainable as a result of mutations in either of these two pathways.

Thus, lessons learned from studying the rare familial cases of colon cancer have illuminated the understanding of the far more common non-familial forms of the disease.

SUMMARY OF CANCER GENETICS

- Rare causes of cancer have enlightened our understanding of common tumors.
- Studies of RNA transforming viruses have led to the discovery of proto-oncogenes that are somatically mutated (and dominantly activated) in many forms of cancer.
- Studies of cancer families have led to the identification of tumor suppressor genes, also showing frequent inactivation (of both alleles) in sporadic cases of similar type.
- Cancer is, in general, a multi-step pathway requiring the accumulation of mutations in several proto-oncogenes or tumor suppressor genes. This process can be potentially accelerated if a DNA repair gene is hit.

GENE THERAPY

·

The goal of gene therapy is to add, repair, or block the expression of genes in the treatment of inherited, as well as non-inherited, diseases. The molecular chaperone used to deliver the therapeutic gene, whether it be a virus or a synthetic chemical, is termed the "vector."

SOMATIC VERSUS GERMLINE GENE THERAPY

It is possible to permanently modify the germline of experimental animals, such as mice, through transgenic methods that add genes or targeted homologous recombination methods that "knock out" and replace genes. In theory, it should be possible to do the same in people.

However, it is important to emphasize that all contemporary gene therapy protocols in humans are aimed at manipulating the genome of somatic cells in selected tissues. No one is yet advocating the modification of germ cells. Thus, the effects of the therapy are planned to be limited to the individual undergoing treatment and are not designed to introduce potentially heritable genetic modifications.

EX VIVO VERSUS IN VIVO GENE THERAPY

In ex vivo gene therapy, the cells to be modified are first removed from the patient, genetically modified in tissue culture, then returned to the patient. Methods of in vivo gene therapy attempt to treat the patient with a gene delivery vehicle that will directly modify the genome of the target cells; in the idealized case, the vector would simply be injected into the patient's vein, injected intramuscularly, or inhaled and then deliver the gene to the appropriate target organ.

GENE THERAPY STRATEGIES

GENE ADDITION

Autosomal recessive and sex-linked recessive inherited diseases typically result from an insufficiency of the normal gene product. Gene therapy protocols designed to treat autosomal recessive diseases are, therefore, aimed at adding a functional copy of the gene to cells that normally express the defective gene.

GENE BLOCKING THERAPIES AND GENE REPAIR

In contrast to recessive diseases, autosomal dominant diseases would not be amenable to simple addition of the correct gene. After all, one of the alleles present in the cell is already normal. The normal allele is insufficient to prevent the disease, because the disease allele expresses a protein that either interferes (dominant negative effects) with the protein product of the normal allele, or else, has a novel function (toxic gain of function). In this situation, the goal of gene therapy is either to extinguish expression from the mutant allele or to correct the mutation.

Antisense

One method for negating gene expression involves the introduction of a single stranded DNA, RNA, or even synthetic nucleic acid derivative that is complementary to the sequence of the targeted gene. This complementary "antisense" nucleic acid can then bind to the single stranded mRNA transcribed from the targeted gene to create a double stranded molecule that is no longer able to be translated.

Ribozymes

Another approach for negating gene expression is to take advantage of catalytic RNAs. Some RNA sequences, typically from introns, have been determined to have catalytic activity that allows them to enzymatically function (hence the name ribozyme), often as a nuclease capable of cutting other RNA species. Ribozymes can be engineered to achieve specificity through complementary basepairing to the targeted mRNA and then deliver their "warhead" of adjacent catalytically active RNA sequence that will destroy the targeted transcript.

Targeted homologous recombination

Targeted homologous recombination is used to repair a defective gene. The principle is to introduce a gene's normal DNA sequence as a template from which the cellular machinery normally active in DNA repair and meiotic recombination is tricked into replacing and, thereby, repairing a defective sequence in the cell. Although the low efficiency of this process is a current impediment to its successful deployment in clinical trials, it is perhaps the most aesthetic—and theoretically safest—of all emerging gene therapy technologies.

GENE DELIVERY VEHICLES

There are two major types of gene delivery vehicles, those based on viruses, and those that are not, relying instead, on physical chemical properties to deliver DNA into cells.

NONVIRAL METHODS

Liposomes

Most of the nonviral methods of gene delivery are modifications of procedures originally developed for the in vitro transfection of DNA in tissue culture cells. Nonviral methods have also been employed, however, in trials of in vivo gene therapy. The majority of effort in nonviral gene therapy is focused on the development of liposomes. A liposome is an ambipathic molecule capable of binding to DNA and incorporating it into a lipid bilayer, which facilitates endocytic entry of the DNA into cells. Liposomal and other nonviral methods of gene therapy efficiently transfect many established cultured "cell lines," but are not so effective at delivery of DNA to cultured primary human cells—as would be required for ex vivo gene therapy—and are even less efficient at transfecting cells when applied in vivo.

Another concern with nonviral methods is that once the therapeutic DNA has entered the nucleus of the target cell, it "integrates" into the genome only exceptionally rarely. (By integration, we mean that the foreign gene inserts itself into the target cell genome by actual physical breakage and re-ligation of DNA.) Thus, unless an effort is made to supply the therapeutic gene with genetic elements that allow it to autonomously replicate (much like a virus), then, as the target cell divides, the therapeutic DNA—if not already degraded by nucleases that recognize it as foreign or damaged—will segregate with only one of the daughter cells and become progressively diluted with each subsequent mitosis.

Naked DNA

At some low level of efficiency, even "naked DNA" directly injected into tissue, especially muscle, may lead to low level transient expression of the therapeutic gene. For some situations this may be desirable. One potential application is DNA-based vaccination—in which it may be preferable to have the host cell generate the foreign protein antigen directly rather than deliver the purified antigen or disabled infectious agent, as is the case with most conventional vaccination methods.

VIRAL METHODS

Perhaps more promising are methods of gene therapy based on viral vectors. The process of using a virus to carry a foreign gene into a cell is referred to as transduction. Several different viral vectors are currently in development.

Retroviruses

These were historically the first viral vectors contemplated for gene therapy. Retroviral vectors are replication defective and require in vitro co-cultivation with "helper" viruses to produce intact viral particles. Because they are replication incompetent, there is less concern that the vector will reproduce and infect either unintended target tissues in the host (such as the testes or ovaries and thereby, risk germline transmission) or spread infectiously to other people who contact the gene therapy patient. Because of the packaging constraints of the virion, retroviral vectors cannot accept a therapeutic gene greater than about 6 to 8 kilobases in DNA length. The modified retroviral genome and therapeutic gene integrate into the host cell genome at random locations. This ensures that there will be reasonably prolonged expression and that the therapeutic gene will be stablely mitotically transmitted as the target cell divides. A potential disadvantage is that there is a risk that the retrovirus will disrupt a gene at the site of insertion and lead to either its loss of activity or inappropriate expression. (If it were a tumor suppressor gene, or proto-oncogene, one could imagine that this may lead to cancer.) So far, these concerns have been largely theoretical and have not resulted in known disease in animal or human trials, however. Retroviruses can only infect dividing cells. As only a small percentage of cells in any somatic tissue is dividing at any particular time, this is one limitation to their efficiency for in vivo gene therapy protocols. Retroviruses are most commonly contemplated for use in ex vivo gene therapy protocols attempting to modify hematopoietic stem cells from the bone marrow.

Adenovirus

Adenoviral vectors are modified from cold viruses that normally infect the human respiratory tract. A great advantage of adenoviral vectors is that "high titer" stocks can be easily prepared. This means that large numbers of infectious particles carrying the therapeutic gene can be concentrated in small volumes, leading to efficient infection of the targeted cells. Adenovirus does not integrate into the host genome and can infect non-dividing cells, unlike retroviruses. Unfortunately, however, adenovirus induces a significant host inflammatory and immune response, and thus far, expression of the therapeutic gene has proven to be of short duration. Adenoviral vectors have found application in both ex vivo and in vivo gene therapy trials where high levels of transient expression of the therapeutic gene is desired. The size limitations of the therapeutic gene that can be packaged with adenovirus is currently about the same as retroviruses. Nevertheless, the adenoviral genome is significantly larger than retroviruses, and efforts are under way to develop newer adenoviral vectors that will accept larger amounts of exogenous DNA.

Adeno-associated virus (AAV)

AAV is a single stranded DNA virus that requires adenovirus as a helper virus to productively infect cells. The native AAV has an unusual property in that it tends to integrate into the targeted human cell genome fairly specifically at a certain locus on chromosome 19. However, AAV modified for use as a vector has lost this site specificity. At present, AAV has attracted much attention for both ex vivo and particularly, in vivo, gene therapy because it appears to provide prolonged and moderately high levels of expression of the therapeutic gene. Its single stranded genome may also make it valuable in gene replacement strategies that make use of targeted homologous recombination. The size limit of the gene that can be packaged is somewhat smaller than that which can be delivered by retroviruses and adenovirus.

Other vectors

Other viruses are being investigated for their potential use in gene therapy applications and include lentiviruses such as HIV (that appear capable of infecting non-dividing cells) and herpesviruses and poxviruses (that may have the capacity to deliver extraordinarily large genes).

EXAMPLES OF CLINICAL APPLICATIONS OF GENE THERAPY

An initial consideration of gene therapy must address the packaging size limits of the vector. Some human genes are immense, such as the dystrophin gene, in which mutations cause Duchenne's muscular dystrophy, and whose length is about one million basepairs. Fortunately, many human mRNAs are smaller than this, and, for still other genes, including dystrophin, functional derivative "mini-genes" can often be prepared.

The following are some examples of gene therapy protocols that have addressed the treatment of inherited and acquired human diseases.

CYSTIC FIBROSIS

Several protocols have considered the potential in vivo genetic therapy of cystic fibrosis. Many protocols have focused on the use of aerosolized and inhaled adenovirus and liposomal preparations to deliver the native CFTR "cDNA" (DNA copy of the mRNA) to the respiratory epithelium.

SICKLE CELL ANEMIA

One gene therapy approach to sickle cell disease involves ex vivo transduction of the erythrogenic precursor cells of the bone marrow with retroviral vectors encoding a normal beta globin gene. The genetically modified cells are then returned to the patient.

HEMOPHILIA B

Current in vivo gene therapy approaches to the treatment of hemophilia B are investigating the potential of AAV to deliver and enable long-term expression of the factor IX blood clotting component by hepatocytes.

CANCER

One approach for cancer treatment involves "suicide" gene therapy. In several trials, typically, a herpesvirus has been used to deliver a herpesvirus thymidine kinase gene to brain tumors. This strategy takes advantage of the fact that the anti-herpes viral agents, acyclovir and ganciclovir, are specifically phosphorylated to toxic inhibitors of DNA replication by the viral, but not the cellular, thymidine kinase. Thus, tumor cells specifically infected by vectors carrying a herpesvirus thymidine kinase gene may be subsequently selectively killed by administering acyclovir or ganciclovir to the patient. Another approach contemplated for cancer treatment is to deliver normally functioning copies of p53, RB, or other tumor suppressor genes to tumor cells that have undergone somatic mutation in order to restore more normal cellular growth characteristics.

THE FUTURE OF GENE THERAPY

Finally, a cautionary note. Gene therapy has yet to become a routine and is only now beginning to emerge from a strictly experimental stage of development. Most gene therapy trials to date have focused more on investigating potential feasibility and safety rather than having been designed to induce benefit. In fact, there are diminishingly few trials—if any—that have offered convincing evidence of clinical benefit to the patients who have been treated. On the other hand, there is no reason to doubt that technological barriers to its success will ultimately be surmounted.

I N D E X

Page numbers followed by *f* indicate figures; numbers followed by *t* indicate tables.

Familial adenomatous polyposis
(FAP), 125–126
Fanconi anemia, 130
FAP (familial adenomatous polypo-
sis), 125–126
FGFR (fibroblast growth factor recep-
tor) gene, 46
Fibrillin gene, 18
Fibroblast growth factor receptor
(FGFR) gene, 46
FISH (fluorescence in situ hybridiza-
tion), 89–91, 100
Fitness, 48
Fluorescence in situ hybridization
(FISH), 89–91, 100
FMR1 gene, 71
Founder effect, 49–50, 52, 66–67, 127
Fragile X syndrome, 70, 82*f*
fragile sites, 70–71
full mutation, 72–73, 76–78, 76–78*f*
inheritance of, 72–78
molecular basis of fragile X, 71–72
premutation carrier, 71–75, 73–75*f*
Frame shift mutation, 49
Friedreich's ataxia, 82, 82*f*

G banding, 86, 87*t*, 88*f*
G protein, 45
"Gain of function" mutation, 17, 119
Gene:
definition of, 4–5
structure of, 7
Gene addition, 135
Gene amplification, 119
Gene blocking therapy, 135–136
Gene delivery:
nonviral methods, 136
viral methods, 137–138
Gene repair, 135–136
Gene therapy, 133–139
clinical applications of, 138–139
ex vivo, 134
future of, 139
germline, 134

goal of, 134
in vivo, 134
somatic, 134
strategies for, 134–138
suicide genes, 139
Genetic disease, 1–2
Genetic recombination. *See* Recombi-
nation
Genetic testing:
direct, 53–54
haplotype analysis, 63–68, 63–64*f*
indirect testing, 54–63
Genotype, 4
Germline gene therapy, 134
Germline mosaicism, 44–45, 44*f*, 47
Glucose-6-phosphate dehydrogenase
(G6PD)deficiency, 52
Gonadoblastoma, 94
G6PD (glucose-6-phosphate dehydro-
genase) deficiency, 52
Guanine, 5–6

Haldane's rule, 48
Haploid, 8, 10
Haploinsufficiency, 17
Haplotype, 33
Haplotype analysis, 63–68, 63–64*f*
Hardy-Weinberg law, 29–31, 30*f*
Hartwell, Leland, 129
HCG (human chorionic
gonadotropin), 104
Head injury, 107
Hearing loss:
age related, 108–109, 108*f*
predisposition to deafness, 42
Hemizygote, 35
Hemochromatosis, 30–31
Hemoglobin, 51–52
Hemophilia A, 35–40, 36–39*f*
Hemophilia B, gene therapy in, 139
Hereditary nonpolyposis colorectal
cancer (HNPCC), 130–131, 131*f*
Herpesvirus:
as gene delivery vehicle, 138

N O T E S

· N O T E S ·

· N O T E S ·

· N O T E S ·

· N O T E S ·

· N O T E S ·

ISBN 0-07-134500-0

90000